MW01489163

# Impatiently Waiting for Miracles

**Impatiently Waiting for Miracles**
Written by: Abby Gray
Foreword by: Brittany N. Clayborne, MS, PsyD
Edited by: Brenda Cortez and Angie Torvik
Interior Layout: Michael Nicloy

Published by: BC Books, LLC
Franklin, Wisconsin
Brenda E. Cortez, Publisher
bcbooksllc.com
Info@bcbooksllc.com

ISBN: 979-8-9907205-2-7

Printed in the United States of America

Daniella-
   Thank you for your support and
encouragement throughout our journey.
                    ♡
               -Abby

To Reid, Oliver, and Kaylee:

You always have been and always will be worth fighting for.

# Table of Contents

# Foreword

As a heart transplant and cancer survivor and a self-proclaimed "collector of miracles," I am always drawn to stories of perseverance and hope. These stories not only remind me of my own journey but reveal the kinship of a shared tribe—a resilient family of fighters who face life's trials with courage, refusing to surrender and holding fast to their deepest dreams.

After reading *Impatiently Waiting for Miracles*, I knew I had found fellow warriors in Abby and Reid. Their journey is one of modern-day heroics, an emotional, soul-testing odyssey filled with unimaginable setbacks and triumphs. Abby's story of navigating the uncertainty of fertility, grieving each loss along the way, and confronting the fear of losing her husband to liver disease is not for the faint of heart. The physical and emotional toll of infertility, compounded by her husband's diagnosis, transformed every day into an uphill battle. Yet Abby and Reid held onto their love, courage, and superhuman hope as they pursued their dream of building a family, with unwavering support from loved ones by their side.

Through it all, their family and friends became sources of strength, love, and resilience. Abby and Reid allowed their parents, best friends, and even elementary school friends to share in their journey, finding light in the compassion of others on the darkest of days. In their willingness to let others in, Abby and Reid experienced a profound healing that only comes from embracing community in the face of hardship. Their story reminds us that even in life's hardest moments, leaning on others can be a powerful source of comfort and strength— and that we are never truly alone when we let others share our burdens.

What makes their story so profoundly moving is its raw, transparent honesty. Abby's openness is healing for anyone in the midst of their own wait for a miracle, as she reveals not only the pain of endurance but also the quiet strength and unexpected blessings that arise from it.

The Grays' journey is a powerful testament to the grit it takes to hold onto dreams, even when they feel impossibly distant. Abby shares her story not as a tale of tragedy, but as a testament to resilience, faith, and the conviction that struggles are never without purpose. I hope that, as you turn these pages, you find comfort in the depth of their faith, and a reminder that even in the darkest hours, it's always worth waiting for a miracle.

Humbly Submitted,

Brittany N. Clayborne, MS, PsyD

# Trigger warnings & disclaimers

If you are searching for a story that will inspire you and remind you of the strength found in community, you're in the right place. However, I do want to offer a few trigger warnings: this book addresses topics such as chronic illness, pregnancy loss, the loss of loved ones, and mental health struggles. That said, without giving too much away, I can promise it concludes in a way that will leave you feeling uplifted and hopeful despite the emotional journey you'll experience.

This book was published in 2025, and the medical procedures and illnesses discussed occurred between 2014 and 2019. I am confident that, over time, advances in medicine will change how some of these situations are handled. Please understand that I'm sharing our personal experiences as they happened. If you are in similar circumstances, it's always best to seek guidance from a medical professional.

For resources and other books by Abby Gray, please visit abbygraywrites.com.

# Prologue

## Reality Hits

### April 13, 2017

I shivered and wondered whether it was because of the cold air in the hospital waiting room or my own fragile nerves. I looked around at the muted blue shades and tan décor of the second-floor waiting room, which overlooked the hospital's first floor. We were surrounded by other families waiting on their loved ones, and I was grateful I had my mom and my husband's parents beside me.

The four of us attempted to keep the conversation light, but our thoughts were quite heavy.

The longer we sat, the larger the knot in my stomach felt. My husband, Reid, had gone through these procedures before—several of them—but this time, it was taking too long.

I tried to keep my composure and hide the immense worry I felt through my entire body. I really needed to pee, but I couldn't go now. What if they came to give us an update and I wasn't here?

I massaged the spot behind my left thumb. I heard that helps with nerves before public speaking, so maybe it would help now. I shifted in my chair, trying to get comfortable but truthfully wanting to be anywhere else.

Then, a hospital volunteer called for the family of Timothy Reid Gray, and when we stood, she escorted us to a private waiting room. The room was just off of the main waiting area, and the plaque on the outside read "Family Waiting Room." It was much smaller, with only six chairs. I immediately felt more confined. My heart sank. This can't be good.

After what felt like forever, a nurse finally walked into the room. "Mrs. Gray? The doctor is ready to talk with you now." She tried to remain as stoic as possible, but I could sense the seriousness of the imminent conversation. I wanted to bring my mother-in-law back with me because I knew I wouldn't want to relay this information myself, but only one of us could go back. For a split second, I debated sending her instead. Was I ready to hear what the doctor had to say? Did I have the strength to absorb this information and then walk back out to tell our family? *Buck up, Abby. You can do hard things.*

Dr. Reddy met me at the front of the recovery area, which he had never done before. Every other time, I was allowed to go back to Reid's bedside and see him, and then the doctor would give us both an update. But this time, they weren't allowing me to go back and see him yet. *The news must be bad,* I thought, *if the doctor wouldn't even tell me in front of my husband, the patient.*

Reid and I knew this doctor well. He had been a great support to us, and we trusted him. He was always a straight shooter, and I expected this time would be no different.

I sensed that this information would change the course of our lives together.

We stood in the open area, leaning on the front edge of the reception desk. I looked around at the drawn curtains of the recovery bays, wondering if my husband was behind one of those curtains.

Dr. Reddy asked the nurse for a piece of paper from the printer nearby, which she grabbed quickly. On that paper, he drew bile ducts and a liver. I watched closely as he scribbled inside the bile ducts to show me exactly where Reid had major blockages instead of open passageways into his liver.

While I appreciated this visual, I just wanted him to skip to the point. *What are we dealing with here? How bad is this, and what does it mean for our future?*

Reid's disease had progressed significantly after only a few years of us thinking *maybe* he would need a liver transplant **someday.**

Dr. Reddy finally imparted the dreaded words. "It's time to call the transplant center and start the process to get him listed."

Tears filled my eyes as I stood there trying to absorb every word that came out of his mouth so I could relay it to our family and Reid. My head was already spinning as I thought about what the transplant process would require and questioned how we could be having this conversation about my 31-year-old husband.

Then, the doctor wrote a percentage at the top of that same piece of paper. **90+%.** He stared at me intently and said, "90+%. This is Reid's chances of developing cancer in his bile ducts – cholangiocarcinoma – if he doesn't receive a liver transplant soon."

I knew his health had declined, but I still wasn't mentally prepared for the gut punch Dr. Reddy had just thrown my way. This was not a routine spyglass procedure (an endoscopic procedure to closely examine the bile ducts in his liver). We were here in the hospital because, for the second time in a month, Reid had to be hospitalized due to excruciating pain in his abdomen. His body was trying to fight off a cholangitis infection that had developed in the bile ducts of his liver, and the pain was unbearable. Reid's liver was trying to kill him.

Reid and I had been married for three years, and we were trying (with difficulty) to start a family. Now, we were told he needed to be listed for a liver transplant, and he also had a 90+% chance of developing cancer if he didn't get that transplant soon.

I tried to focus on all the information the doctor had just blindsided me with while also trying to keep my composure. I needed to deliver this news to our family, but how? How could this be where we were in our life together? Lately, we had been so focused on creating a family together, but now I questioned whether Reid would even be around to be part of that family.

I wiped the tears streaming down my cheeks and thanked Dr. Reddy for the information. He hugged me and advised me to share the news with our family in the waiting room. Once I passed on the dreaded news, I could head back to see Reid as he was still waking up from the anesthesia.

I began walking back to the waiting room, but before I could get there, my body pushed me against the stark white wall of the hallway, and I burst into tears. I stood there trying to stop the tears and urging myself to keep walking. I knew our family was waiting. They were just on the other side of those sterile double doors, and I didn't want them to hear my cries. By this point, I figured they had a hunch it wasn't good news, so I knew every second I kept them waiting was excruciating for them, too. I gathered myself, or so I thought.

I walked into the private waiting room and tried to shut the door. This news shouldn't be shared with an open door just off a crowded waiting room.

My father-in-law's chair prevented me from closing the door to the already cramped room, but I couldn't even mutter the words to ask him to move. Instead, I just motioned with my hand. I then realized I was holding my breath, trying not to cry, and as soon as I opened my mouth, no words came out. Only sobs. *Pull it together, Abby*, I thought. *This is only making it harder on them. You've got to get through this, and then you can have your breakdown. They need to know what you know.*

My mom grabbed a chair for me and placed it in front of them so the three of them could see my face. I looked at my mother-in-law, whose tear-filled eyes pleaded for the information. She had pulled her strawberry-red hair into a low ponytail, and the worry had obviously taken over her entire body. My mom, wearing a t-shirt instead of her usual cute outfit, watched me closely, and I felt as though she was silently trying to send me her strength to help me through this. The room was quiet as I wiped tears from my eyes and took a few deep breaths to calm my nervous system.

I finally pulled it together enough to speak and started with, "Reid is out of the procedure and okay at the moment. But…" All the information Dr. Reddy shared with me poured out as I tried to remember every detail. My mother-in-law, Tinker, had been a medical researcher for many years. She usually asks many questions, so I wanted to ensure I answered as much as possible when explaining. My numb body switched into auto-pilot as I continued sharing the grim details.

My mom reached for the tissue box on the table beside her and passed out tissues to each person.

I could see the disbelief in my mother-in-law's face and empathized with her reluctance to believe the news I was sharing. My head then turned toward my father-in-law. He had his head down, and I could see the tears slowly streaming down his face.

When I finished sharing the doctor's information, we all sat there in silence, stunned, not knowing what to do with it.

*What else was there to say? When was the right time to get up and see Reid in recovery?* My heart ached to be with him after his procedure, but I also didn't want to share this information with him until he was fully awake. Every other time he'd had a procedure,

I would have to repeat the doctor's update several times as the anesthesia wore off. Repeating those details would have torn me apart.

After sharing the procedure results with our family, and we had our time to shed tears, I went to see Reid. As I walked back through the double sterile doors, I leaned on that same wall to catch my breath. I needed to put on a brave face. I don't hide my emotions well, so I knew Reid would know the results weren't good by the look on my face.

I went to the recovery bay and pulled back the curtain to see the nurse leaning over his bed, asking how he was feeling. Reid was groggy, and it was apparent he had just woken up. I gave him a half-smile and felt we somehow had an unspoken agreement. He didn't ask, and I didn't tell. He just knew. He didn't know fully, but he knew.

I sat in the guest chair beside his bed as the nurse looked at me and asked, "Dr. Reddy talked to you, right?" I nodded to her and sucked in my breath to keep from breaking down again.

Reid looked at me as if to ask for an update, so I told him, "The procedure went well, but it just took a little longer. I will update you more as soon as you can remember."

When the results were good, I always shared them right away. I didn't mind repeating myself as many times as I needed to while he came out of his haze. "All is good, no major progress. We'll be back in a few months for another procedure," I usually respond. That wasn't the case this time.

We sat silently as I tried to think of something else to say. Reid was quiet to avoid being laughed at. Because of his illnesses, he underwent regular colonoscopies and endoscopies and is always entertaining with his funny remarks while coming down from anesthesia.

Once, after a colonoscopy, he mixed up which procedure he had just had, telling me, "My throat doesn't even hurt this time!"

I belly laughed and responded, "That's great since they went in the other end today."

After another endoscopy, he proudly told the nurse, "I dreamt I was one of the Avengers!"

When she inquired about his superpowers, he shook his head disappointingly and said, "I wasn't a very good superhero."

After quite a few procedures together, he had enough self-control to stop himself before saying things that would make me and the nurse laugh at his expense. Instead, he would give me a "thumbs up" with a knowing look, which he did then. I swear the look was, "I refuse to give you more ammunition." It made me laugh a little.

We are those people who are constantly joking, no matter the situation, so I tried to keep it light-hearted. But this time, my heart was not light.

He finally looked at me and said, "Okay, I think I'm ready to hear it. You may have to repeat it, but I'm mostly aware." I honestly can't tell you how he responded when I told him the news because my head was now in a complete fog. Reid is pretty stoic about health stuff, so I imagine he didn't have a big reaction. He took the information in and sat with it.

I tried to focus on the things I could control. I'm a "doer" and like to have control over the situation, but this was unchartered territory. I thought of what I could focus on, such as calling the transplant center. I also needed to share the latest news with our support system – at this point, we had come to rely heavily on them.

After what felt like forever sitting in an uncomfortable hospital guest chair, Reid's nurse said they were moving him back up to his hospital room soon, and I could walk with them. I texted his mom to tell them they could start heading that way, and we'd see them back in his room.

On the way up to his hospital room, we passed by my mom, sitting in a small waiting area just outside of Reid's room. She was on the phone and crying. When she looked up and saw the nurse pushing

Reid's hospital bed, I could see her panic. She attempted to hide her tears, but it was too late.

Then, we met Reid's parents in his room. As we walked in, they frantically tried to wipe the tears streaming down their faces since they weren't sure how much he knew. I looked at them and said, "He knows." I did not want them to feel like they had to hold back.

Once the nurse situated Reid's hospital bed into the empty spot in the room, his parents went to his side. The room was still dark from when we left earlier that morning, and the only light was shining through the large windows that lined one wall. Somehow, the room felt smaller than it had just that morning.

As Reid lay in his hospital bed absorbing the unwelcomed outcome of his procedure, my father-in-law, a mighty football coach, went to his side and held his 6'8" son and cried. That picture of a father's love and pain is forever etched in my mind. He wanted so badly to protect his son and remove the hurt and hardship.

Reid tried to hold back his tears as the news sank in. His parents stood by his bedside as I sat down on the couch. This unfamiliar feeling had me crawling in my skin, and I didn't know what to do. The room became silent since none of us knew what to say at that moment.

Reid's parents then offered to give us time alone to process our future fate together. As soon as they left, I crawled into bed with my husband, and we both let go of the tears we were choking down. I whispered to him, "We will be okay. We will figure this out."

Both of us knew the fight ahead would be a big one. We had yet to learn what the future would bring and whether our dream of building a family would ever become a reality.

When Reid's initial diagnosis of liver disease, primary sclerosing cholangitis, was given, we felt a lot of uncertainty surrounding what life with this disease would look like for him. Maybe one day, he would need a liver transplant, but maybe he wouldn't. We knew that with this disease (and his simultaneous diagnosis of ulcerative colitis), he was much more likely to develop cancer, either in his bile ducts or in his colon.

After we wrapped our heads around the news together, I found my in-laws and my mom standing in the hallway just outside his room. Their tear-streaked faces and red eyes couldn't hide their anguish.

I asked them to go sit with Reid since I needed to start making phone calls. The initial shock had worn off, and I had pivoted into "action" mode. I needed our troops to rally, and I needed to figure out how to save my husband.

This was not going to be how things ended.

# Chapter 1

# Our Beginning

## 2011–2012

I dated my share of guys before I found my wonderful husband. One night in 2011, I went out with some friends, complaining about the most recent guy I had been on a few dates with.

One of the girls insisted, "I have a guy for you! He's an engineer, really nice, cute, and super tall!"

I'm 5' 9", so I've always preferred taller guys, but Maria, the girl trying to set me up, was maybe 5'2", so I thought, *everyone is tall to you; we'll see about this.*

She asked, "Can I give him your number?"

I responded, "Sure, but I doubt he calls." There had been (a lot of) alcohol consumed that night, so I wasn't sure she'd even remember to reach out to him.

I had never been on a blind date before but wasn't opposed to it. I figured it would take a lot of guts to call a woman you had never met and ask her out, so I thought, *we'll see if it ever happens.*

A few weeks passed, and I completely forgot about the conversation.

Three weeks later, I missed a call from an area code I didn't recognize. The person didn't leave a message, so I assumed it must have been a sales call. The next day, I got another call from that same number. This time, I answered, ready to tell them I wasn't interested.

When I answered, the guy on the other end said, "Hi, Abby. This is Reid Gray, Maria's friend."

"Who??" I snapped, still thinking it was a salesperson—poor guy.

He responded, "Um, yeah, this is Reid Gray. Maria gave me your number."

It clicked. "Oh! Hi Reid. I'm sorry, I thought you were a salesperson."

In my defense, I don't even remember her telling me his name, and he took THREE WEEKS to call me. He asked me to join him for "drinks or dinner" the following Tuesday. I accepted, and we agreed on a time and place.

We met at a restaurant in City Centre at 7 PM. Before our date, I Facebook-stalked him so I would know a little about this stranger I planned to meet up with, or at least know what he looked like. I also sent his Facebook profile and phone number to some of my friends, just in case I went missing.

I wore a pair of my tallest wedges to test the "super tall" theory. Reid was sitting on a bench just inside the restaurant's front door. When I came in, he stood to greet me. He had obviously checked out my Facebook profile since he recognized me immediately. As he stood, I realized Maria wasn't lying when she described him as "super tall." I think 6'8" qualifies.

He wore an Under Armour polo shirt, jeans, and cowboy boots. I would later learn that the cowboy boots were one of his first purchases after moving to Texas a few years ago. He had short strawberry blonde hair which he spiked at the front, and the light coming in the door from the evening sun made his blue eyes shine even brighter. His warm smile embraced me with comfort, although I sensed his heart pounding and figured he was trying to hide his nerves. I had been quite nervous, but somehow, his nervousness calmed me.

We sat on the restaurant's patio, which I now know is not typical for him as Reid hates the Texas heat and eating amongst the bugs. But he did his best to go with the flow for our first date. Plus, the patio was much quieter, which made it easier to carry on a conversation.

Our "drinks or dinner" date turned into four hours of talking, a couple of drinks, and a full meal. We had a great time and didn't realize how late it was until they started sweeping the floors!

Reid told me he grew up in Indianapolis and had been recruited as an engineer from Purdue University. I am a born-and-raised Texas girl who had no plans to move away from my family, so I asked, "Do you ever plan to return to Indiana?"

He replied, "No, I'm good here in Texas." Whew, okay, we could continue this conversation.

He shared that he is a Chicago Cubs baseball fan. I chuckled because I had just attended an Astros-Cubs game the week before. While at the game, I noticed that even though we were in Minute Maid Park, the Cubs fans were louder and more obnoxious. I wondered secretly if he was one of *those* Cubs fans.

Spoiler alert – he is.

Around 11 PM, we decided to call it a night since the restaurant employees were trying to close around us. He walked me to my car, then slowly leaned in and hugged me. That left me wondering if the date wasn't as good for him since he didn't even try to kiss me. That kiss-less first date left me looking forward to another date and that first kiss even more. We parted ways and agreed we'd hang out again.

Our relationship started a little rocky…from my perspective, not Reid's. Our first few dates were great, but I just wasn't sure if I was ready to spend all my time with this one guy. Don't get me wrong—I thought he was smart, sweet, funny, handsome, and athletic, and we had a great time together. He was a nerd but also really into sports, and he had been a tri-sport athlete in high school.

I had a type-A personality and big aspirations of growing my career in downtown Houston and making connections in the business community. We were opposites in the ways we both needed. Reid had a calmness about him that eased my high-strung personality. He was a numbers guy, and I was a people person. Reid was excellent with money, but I didn't quite understand the importance of a budget. Our personalities balanced each other well, and we were alike in ways that mattered – both sarcastic and joking most of the time, and our core values were aligned.

I just wasn't sure I was ready to settle down. Fortunately, Reid was persistent.

I asked him once, "Why do you want to hang out with me so often?"

He chuckled and said, "I just like you and want to spend time with you. Is that a problem?"

I think I had been enjoying the freedom of single life a little too much before we met, but our love grew over the next several weeks, and we became exclusive. I remember us sitting on the couch one night talking after watching a movie together. I got quiet as I looked at him, and he asked, "What's on your mind?"

I hesitated and replied, "This is so great, I'm just…"

He responded, "Waiting for the other shoe to drop?"

"Yes!" I said with a little too much enthusiasm.

We got along well, and things felt effortless when we were together. But it terrified me that there was some huge red flag I hadn't seen yet. He felt the same way.

A few months after we started dating, I was having a hard time at work and not loving my job anymore. I had spent the last few weeks in tears, not knowing how to fix the frustrations I was dealing with or what to do next. Reid wanted to help and knew I needed a break from work.

He suggested we take a few days off and fly back to his hometown to meet his parents and relax. While I wanted to meet them, I felt my current state of mind wasn't ideal. Also, how could a trip to meet your boyfriend's parents be relaxing?

Despite my hesitations, we flew to Indiana to spend a couple of days with them, and it turned out to be just what I needed. I fell in love with his parents and saw myself fitting into his family. We sat on their screened-in porch in our pajamas each morning, talking. Before we came, his mom had requested a list of my favorite foods and drinks, so she made sure to have those items in the house. They didn't have an itinerary while we were there. They only wanted to enjoy our company and let the trip be as relaxing as we needed. We lounged and talked and lounged some more. They also took me to their favorite pizza place.

Meeting Reid's parents, Ric and Tinker, confirmed things for me. And I'm not just saying that because my mother-in-law is proofreading this book!

That week, I began discussing marriage with Reid. I was ready.

He had his own timeline.

Reid had been in a relationship for five years, spanning through high school and college, and thought at the time he would marry her. Their devastating breakup blindsided him. As a result, he had some trust issues and wanted to make sure I wouldn't do the same to him. He had his timeline, I had mine, and we needed to meet in the middle.

I am a strong-willed person and a bit of a control freak, and at that point in my life, all of my decisions had been relatively minor and only affected me: where to live, where to take a job, who to be friends with, what to have for dinner. Being in a relationship meant I needed to make decisions with another person, and I quickly realized just how pushy I was. When Reid and I first started dating, he was a bit (okay, a lot) of a push-over.

One time, when I asked him to do something for me, he told me, "No."

I raised my hand to give him a high-five, and he flinched. I'm not even kidding. I feel the need to say that I have never and would never hit him.

He said, "What are you doing?"

I quipped, "Giving you a high-five. You told me no!"

We each had different styles, communication methods, and baggage from past relationships, just as any new couple does. I was much more direct, while he avoided confrontation. I could be a bit of a pessimist, and he was usually an optimist.

I was more traditional in thinking the guy drives how quickly the relationship moves (but not so traditional that I took up cooking and cleaning, despite my grandma reminding me often that I should). I wanted him to ask me to move in, marry him, etc. I could push my timeline all I wanted, but ultimately, it was up to him, which drove me a little crazy.

Reid is a mechanical engineer for a large oil and gas company. Within six months of dating, he started working off-shore rotations (two weeks on-shore, two weeks off-shore) on an oil rig. I hated it, but it showed me just how much I truly loved him. The saying "absence makes the heart grow fonder" is absolutely true.

Reid was off-shore for our first Thanksgiving and Christmas together, and I spent both holidays sad and missing him. We haven't spent a holiday apart since, thankfully, as his off-shore rotations only lasted about a year.

In between his rotations, we traveled a lot. We went on many road trips with friends and took two international trips together in the first year of dating. One was to China for my job, where we climbed the Great Wall together. He then planned a fantastic trip to Italy for me, my sister, and my sister's boyfriend (now husband). Some friends were convinced he would propose to me in Italy, but I was so sure he wouldn't that I bet a friend $100. I won. Reid wasn't this big romantic gesture kind of guy, so when the time was right, I knew he would do it privately, just the two of us.

We dreamed about all the trips we would take together in the future and learned a lot about each other while traveling.

In February 2012, I moved into the apartment he and his best friend shared.

A few months later, I accepted a new position as a project manager for a small concierge relocation company, with much more flexibility. I had known Julie, the owner, for a little while. She had a kind heart, and it felt right to work for her.

That summer, Reid and I began house shopping. I had my heart set on a specific area of town, close to some of my extended family and my new job. His top priority for the house was to be big enough to create a media room and have space for a pool table. In August, we found a home that met both our criteria, so we bought it. Well, he bought a house for us.

Our new home was a 30-minute drive from where most of our friends lived, but we wanted it to be where everyone came to hang out, so the pool table and media room were set up in the house before we even moved our beds in. The first night in the house, we slept on an air mattress in the media room. We watched *The Usual Suspects*, and I remember dreaming about the memories we'd make in this house together as we lay there.

We loved game nights and hosting our friends and family. Reid is an amazing cook, and our new house had a great open-concept kitchen, which was perfect for entertaining. It also had four bedrooms with plenty of space for kids. In November, we adopted a dog and named him Wrigley (I told you he was one of ***those*** Cubs fans.)

Everything felt perfect. Except where was my damn ring?! Let's get this show on the road! Apparently, it was sitting in the attic, the one place in the house he knew I'd never go. I was too clumsy to be up there, and I proved that years later by stepping through the ceiling the one time I did go up on my own.

December 7th, 2012, Reid proposed in the most perfect way. He loves experimenting in the kitchen and told me about a month earlier he wanted to start trying new recipes for Friday night dinners.

That Friday, he cooked filet with a lobster béarnaise sauce, scalloped potatoes with crab meat, and asparagus. He perfectly cooked the filet, and the potatoes melted in your mouth. After dinner, he asked me to take Wrigley outside while he finished up the dessert.

When I came back in and sat down, he placed a tray in front of me that had two crème brûlée desserts (my FAVORITE, and the reason I was asked to go outside—he didn't want me to hear the blow torch,) two glasses of port wine, and a box with an engagement ring. He dropped to one knee and said, "I love you so much. Will you marry me?"

We were both shaking as I told him YES and pulled him up for a hug.

After we both settled down, he insisted: "You should start calling your people. They're all waiting."

Everyone else already knew his plan, and my mom and best friend were driving circles around our neighborhood, just waiting for my call. Our doorbell rang, and some of our closest friends showed up to celebrate with us, including friends who drove from Dallas to Houston to be there for this huge life event.

Let the wedding planning begin.

# Chapter 2

## Warning Signs

### Spring 2014

We decided on a long engagement. My days were consumed with wedding planning, and I had it down to every little detail. My mom, sister, and best friend are also planners, so they fed into my obsession with making the wedding perfect for us. We picked a wine theme and collected wine bottles for months to use as decorations. My aunt spent hours peeling off wine bottle labels, and my grandma and mom created some beautiful centerpieces.

We held the wedding at a resort overlooking Lake Conroe, about an hour north of Houston, and most of our guests stayed there for the weekend.

When guests arrived at the ceremony, they were greeted with an open bar because we were *those friends* who always wanted to ensure you were having a good time. The rooms where we held both the ceremony and reception overlooked the lake, so we had a gorgeous backdrop for the evening.

I am not a public crier, but when those doors opened for me to walk down the aisle, I nearly lost it. Seeing our friends and family with huge smiles and my groom standing at the end of the aisle took my breath away. I tried so hard not to ugly-cry as I squeezed my dad's arm. I walked down the aisle with tears in my eyes and the biggest smile on my face as I sucked in air, trying to keep the tears in. When we approached the altar, my dad handed me a Kleenex with a trembling hand before shaking Reid's hand and passing me off to him. I was so surprised by how emotional I was that I forgot to hug my dad before he went to sit down.

After the ceremony, our guests headed to the reception hall next door while we took family photos. When they walked into the hall, they were greeted by a DJ playing our favorite tunes, open bars, and some passed appetizers. Each table held a blue, green, and silver centerpiece incorporating wine bottles in different ways. Some were used as candle holders, and some were vases. The guest tables had a photo scavenger hunt and Scrabble tiles with magnets attached to the back that spelled out different love-related words.

Our dinner was so delicious we felt like we were at a fancy steakhouse with 200 of our closest friends and family. Then came the dancing and toasts.

Most of our guests didn't know it, but my dad and I had worked for weeks to practice a choreographed dance for the wedding. We started with the typical father-daughter dance with a waltz to "I loved her first" by Heartland. And then, halfway through, the music came to a screeching halt and changed to a mix that my friend Marisa had created and choreographed for us. Our guests erupted in cheers so loud I couldn't even hear the music at first.

The dance set the tone for a packed dance floor for the rest of the evening. My Mema was even out there dancing with us for most of the night. The dance floor was still packed as our reception ended, so we moved the party to the hotel bar, which was having a karaoke night. It was truly a night that will forever live in my memory.

We went on our honeymoon two months after our wedding, as March was not the best time to visit Santorini, Greece. While I obsessed over the wedding details, Reid had been doing tons of research to plan the perfect honeymoon in the most beautiful location.

Our resort overlooked a vast cliff surrounded by stunning white buildings. We experienced breathtaking sunsets from our balcony in the evening, had breakfast served to us on that balcony each morning, and enjoyed lots of good food and wine. Everyone we encountered during that trip was kind and welcoming as we explored the island each day.

Reid began to complain of a stomachache halfway through the honeymoon. We thought it was all the rich food we had been enjoying and possibly just being off due to travel. That day, we lay on our balcony and napped off and on throughout the day, taking in the amazing views.

The next day, I was ready to get out and explore more. I will admit I wasn't very sympathetic to the fact that he wasn't feeling well. I told him we were on our honeymoon and he should suck it up so we could explore. Yes, I was already proving to be a wonderfully supportive wife. He did as I requested, powered through, and hid his pain as best he could.

Shortly after we got back from our honeymoon, I was awake one night with excruciating stomach pain (Hello, Karma? Is that you?) We ended up going to the ER, and they told me I likely had gastritis (an inflamed stomach lining that causes intense pains at times). The ER doctor prescribed medication to help me with the symptoms and referred me to a gastroenterologist.

Reid went to my doctor's appointment with me a few weeks later. He was scared by how much pain I had been in and wondered if that might be what he had on our honeymoon. The gastroenterologist, Dr. Reddy, was so great that he not only took the time to discuss what was wrong with me but also discussed Reid's stomach issues during our honeymoon.

Reid scheduled a follow-up with Dr. Reddy, and at that follow-up appointment, he was diagnosed with ulcerative colitis (UC). UC is a chronic inflammatory bowel disease that causes inflammation and ulcers in the large intestine.

Once diagnosed, Reid mentioned to the doctor that a few years prior, he was denied life insurance due to high liver enzyme numbers. He had seen a few doctors, but no one could tell him what may be wrong. He felt fine but always wondered why he would have been denied life insurance. That seemed like a big deal, but at that time, he was a 20-something male who didn't invest the time to figure it out.

Dr. Reddy asked lots of questions, ran more tests, and finally deduced that Reid had primary sclerosing cholangitis (PSC). PSC is a rare chronic liver disease in which the bile ducts of the liver become very inflamed and scarred, leading to long-term liver damage.

Okay, maybe I should have been a little more compassionate when he said he didn't feel well on our honeymoon.

Dr. Reddy spent the time explaining both diseases to us. The UC would cause him some major discomfort from time to time, but there were medications Reid could try to manage the symptoms. The goal was to manage the pain and get the disease in remission. He mentioned that dietary changes would also help, but Reid didn't like that suggestion. He would rather take all the medication in the world than give up his favorite foods. However, dietary changes would be worth it if they made him feel better.

PSC was more ambiguous, and we had no clear path forward. The disease is rare, so not a lot of research funds have been dedicated to studying it. From what Dr. Reddy knew, it presented differently in each patient, and there was no real way of knowing how quickly it would progress.

Tests could be done, and medication could be given, but no medication had been proven to slow the progression of the disease. All they could say was it *may* help with his minor symptoms at the time, but maybe not.

There is no known cure for PSC, and the only effective treatment option is a liver transplant. He explained that not everyone who has PSC ends up needing a liver transplant. It just depends on how your body handles the disease. He shared that PSC patients do have more challenges in receiving a liver transplant, but if that time came, we would discuss it more then.

Right then, all we needed to know was Reid *may* need a liver transplant one day. Also, with having both ulcerative colitis and primary sclerosing cholangitis, Reid's chances of developing cancer in the gastrointestinal tract were *significantly* higher than the average person.

Dr. Reddy considered all the information and devised a plan for us. He prescribed medications to help manage the symptoms of both diseases and said Reid would need to have regular monitoring through colonoscopies and endoscopies. We could do nothing else right then except adjust medications as needed and monitor how things progressed.

I left that appointment only hearing: "The worst case scenario is liver transplant or cancer, but you're young and otherwise healthy, so hopefully that's not the case." Doctors live in the worst-case scenarios and must be conscious of the potential outcomes. But in my head, I knew that wouldn't be us. Even if it came to that, it wouldn't be for a long time, so we'd only worry about it if or when it happened.

We were newly married, otherwise healthy, and thoroughly enjoying our life together. How could anything derail that? We had a plan with the doctor, so we're good.

All Reid heard was *transplant* and *cancer*. He is usually the optimistic one of the two of us. Annoyingly optimistic. But not this time. I had my glass half-full, while Reid's was half-empty.

After Reid's appointment, we went to one of our favorite restaurants for breakfast. It caught me off-guard that Reid was so distraught since he usually had to remind me there were different sides to the story. Reid always encouraged me to look at the other perspective if a friend or family member upset me. However, that day, he only saw one perspective: we had just gotten married and were about to go through hell. I refused to see things from his angle. He didn't have a crystal ball revealing a grim future. We would be fine. Why bother stressing over something that hadn't happened yet (and, in my mind, likely wouldn't ever happen)?

We called his parents during breakfast and shared the doctor's report. His mom is a self-proclaimed worrier. I knew she would have the same perspective as Reid, but I hoped she didn't voice that on the call and feed into his internal spiral. I could hear the worry in her voice, but she remained calm. My gut told me that as soon as they hung up, his mom would be doing research of her own to understand what this diagnosis meant for him.

In this situation, I felt that time spent worrying about what *may* happen *one day* was wasted. Anyone who knew me then knew that was not my typical perspective—I was also a worrier. Fortunately, Reid and I have always balanced each other out in that way. We filled in the gaps of what each other needed most, and this time was no different. Our differing opinions always helped us find a middle ground that allowed us to work through things together.

Reid has a very analytical brain and thrives on fact-finding. Over the next few days, he went down the rabbit hole of Dr. Google. He read as much as he could about the diseases, and he and his mom had several conversations about PSC and UC as she dug into her medical research.

My determination clung firmly to the belief that we would be okay. It would be a problem for "future" us. We had our action plan and instructions from the doctor, so there wasn't much to do except wait and see what the future would bring.

# Chapter 3

## And Then Comes Baby...Maybe?

### Fall 2014 – Spring 2015

A few months after Reid's diagnosis, I convinced him it was time to build our family. If you had asked me my ideal timeline after college graduation, I planned to be married by 25 and start having kids a year or two later. At 28 and only recently married, I was already behind. I wanted to have as much control over the timeline as possible, but I would soon be reminded that the control was not mine.

My mom had suffered two pregnancy losses before having me and my sister, and she had always been very open with us about her struggles to conceive. I just assumed I would be in the same boat.

Reid had some significant hesitations about starting a family once he learned about the diseases he had. While he didn't voice this to me at the time, he was terrified we would have kids, and then he would become extremely ill and leave me a single mom. He fought me on trying to get pregnant, but I assumed it was just the typical male reaction of never feeling *ready* for that responsibility. He stuffed down his worries, and we pressed forward.

Nine long months and what felt like hundreds of pregnancy tests later, I went to get a spray tan the day before my cousin's wedding. I stood there while the technician was spraying me, and all of a sudden, I felt super lightheaded. I had to sit down as I thought I would pass out.

My friend Amy was with me, and she knew we had been trying to conceive. She immediately said, "Abby, you're pregnant!" *No way. Please don't get my hopes up,* I thought. I had cried **every. single. time.** I got my period over the last nine months. I had convinced myself our only hope of conceiving was with the help of a fertility specialist.

The following morning, I took a pregnancy test. I waited until Reid left for work so he wouldn't see the breakdown I would have when the test came up negative. But there it was: a faint line. I stood in our bathroom, still in a t-shirt and underwear, staring at the test in my hand. I put my hand over my mouth and just started shaking my head. *No way. Am I imagining this?* I dug under my bathroom sink to find two more tests, peed on those, and then stared at them. I was still in disbelief that they were positive.

I threw on some pants, a bra, and flip-flops and got in my car. I had to go to the drugstore for more tests. I needed more proof. I marched into the drugstore and bee-lined for the pregnancy tests. *Was four enough? Yeah, I think that will do.* As the cashier rang up the $30 worth of tests, I wanted to tell her. I wanted to tell everyone.

Seven tests and seven double lines later, I couldn't deny it. I was pregnant.

When I decide to do something, I go all in. So, as soon as we stopped birth control several months before, I became obsessed with how we would share the news with our parents when we learned we were pregnant. I had an entire secret Pinterest board dedicated to it. You couldn't just announce, "I'm pregnant!" In my mind, it had to be done in a big, elaborate way, or you had to buy a special gift. I had wanted to do this type of special announcement for so many years. Whenever I saw a new, unique way someone announced their pregnancy on social media, I'd tuck that idea away for potential future use. My announcement would not be boring; it had to be planned and pre-purchased.

Months before seeing those two pink lines, I ordered gifts for our parents to receive the day I finally got a positive pregnancy test. Reid's parents still lived in Indiana, but they had recently been to Houston to see us. I handed my mother-in-law a wrapped gift when we took them to the airport for their flight home. I told her to hold onto it and that I would call and tell her when to open it. I also had gifts tucked away in my closet for my parents. I had all the bases covered.

After my mad dash to the pharmacy for more tests, I called Reid to tell him the good news. He would tell you I actually called my friend Amy first to tell her she was right. I think he's still bitter about that. But we were finally pregnant! I then called my OB-GYN and made an appointment for later that afternoon.

They did a blood draw at the appointment, but I wouldn't have the results until Monday since it was Friday. It didn't matter because I knew what they'd tell me on Monday—I was pregnant. What more was there to it? Either you're pregnant, or you're not. My seven pregnancy tests were all the proof I needed.

They did a pelvic exam, and then the doctor took me back to his office to talk. He took out his little chart and told me according to my last menstrual cycle, my due date was Christmas Day. *Noooooooooooo!!!* I thought. *But wait, it doesn't matter what the due date is. We are pregnant. That's all that matters.*

The doctor and I discussed what to expect regarding care and monitoring the pregnancy, and then he said they would call me on Monday with the results of my bloodwork.

That night was my cousin's wedding, and most of my family would be attending. We got all dressed up and were excited to celebrate with them, knowing we were finally(!) pregnant. As I put on my dress, I turned in the mirror and looked at my stomach. I couldn't wait to have an adorable bump there.

Most conventional advice tells you not to announce a pregnancy early but rather keep it secret until you are into the second trimester, "just in case." I'm not very conventional, and I also don't keep secrets well or really at all. Screw conventional advice.

On the way to the wedding, the same day we learned we were pregnant, we called Reid's parents and asked them to open the gift we had sent them home with. Tinker said, "Okay…" as she went to find the wrapped gift she had tucked away and told Ric we were on the phone. We both had our phones on speakerphone, and I held mine between Reid and me as he drove us to the wedding.

Tinker opened the angel and read the inscription out loud, "Grandmas are angels on earth." We then shared, "We're pregnant!" Reid's mom loved and collected angels, so I picked this out, especially for her. They were excited and agreed that Christmas would be extra special this year, as Reid's sister, Sarah, was also expecting. There would be two new grandbabies to celebrate.

Once at the wedding reception, Reid and I asked my dad to come to our car with us after we finished dinner because we had a present for him. He opened the "This guy is going to be a Grandpa" (with two thumbs pointing up) shirt that I had wrapped for him, and he burst into tears. What is it about men crying that makes me that much more emotional? I started laughing and crying simultaneously and gave him a big hug. He squeezed me tight as he tried to stop the tears, and I knew I'd remember that moment forever. My sister, Megan, stood there with us as well (of course, I had called her that morning just after I found out), tears in her eyes.

The next day, we planned to go out of town to visit a very close friend of mine for her birthday. We'd be driving right by my mom's house, so I called to tell her we were stopping by for a minute with a surprise. She collected the Willow Tree figurines, so I bought and wrapped up the "Grandmother" figurine for her. She opened it and said, "Thank you!"

"Look at the box," I told her. I knew she didn't realize which figurine I had just given her.

"Grandmother?" She read and looked at me with her eyes wide.

I nodded my head and said, "Yes! We're pregnant!!"

Tears filled her eyes, and she gave me a big hug. She knew we had wanted to be pregnant for months and was so happy for us. Finally, things were coming together, and I could experience these special moments I had dreamed of for so long.

I took the book *What to Expect When You're Expecting* for the road trip, which I had purchased months prior. As we drove, I read about how to care for myself and this baby. We stopped for healthy snacks, and I drank lots of water to stay hydrated. I became hyper-focused on the fact that I was pregnant.

When Monday arrived, I frequently checked my phone, hoping for a call from the doctor's office. When the call finally came in around 4 PM, I was on my way to a meeting on the other side of town. The nurse said, "Your bloodwork shows you're pregnant, but your hCG level (the hormone that shows how far along you are in pregnancy) is low. It may be earlier in your pregnancy than we thought... or something could be wrong. You might be having a miscarriage."

***Miscarriage???*** *No way. This can't be happening.*

We were finally pregnant after nine months of trying. *We can't lose this baby.*

"We want you to come in tomorrow morning for more bloodwork. That will allow us to see how your levels are increasing," she continued, unaware of my internal spiral. She explained they would need to see the hCG increase substantially for this to be a viable pregnancy.

I took the next exit on the freeway, turned my car around, and headed home. I didn't know what to do with myself, but I knew I needed to be home with my husband. I called Reid and told him the news as he was driving home from work. Then I called my mom, my best friend, and my sister. Everyone assured me I wasn't having a miscarriage yet, and the doctor's office was only warning me that it may be possible. My breath quickened, my stomach tightened, and I felt I had no control over the outcome. *Did they seriously expect me to sit and wait for more bloodwork after that call??*

Things remained stable, and my hCG continued to rise for the next week and a half. The level remained right *below* the safe range, but it was still increasing at a fairly even rate, so the outlook seemed optimistic. We went in for our first ultrasound, and they told us it could still be very early, so we may not see anything.

The nurse angled the screen towards her, but we could still see it. She inserted the transvaginal ultrasound wand and found my uterus.

"I don't see much yet. It may just be too early," the nurse said. "There's a small little spot right here (she points to the screen) that may be your baby, but it's unclear yet."

I sighed and looked at Reid. Of course, we couldn't have a straightforward answer today—more waiting.

"Let's check out your fallopian tubes to confirm all is okay there," the nurse said. She moved the wand around and studied the screen. She zoomed in on a spot on my left fallopian tube.

"Have you ever had cysts?" She asked.

"No! Do I have one now?" I barked back.

She studied the screen a little longer and replied, "Maybe. I'm not sure what that is. It's small, so hopefully, it will resolve on its own.

We'll keep an eye on it; there's nothing to worry about right now."

She removed the wand and took off her gloves. I sat up and readjusted the sheet covering my bottom half. "So that's it? We wait and see?" I asked.

"Yes, we'll schedule you for another ultrasound in a couple of weeks, and by then, we'll be able to see more. Just continue with bloodwork for now, and we'll see you back soon," she replied as if it was just another day in the office.

After she left the room, I dressed and headed to the reception desk to schedule a follow-up appointment.

Despite the uncertainty of that appointment, I needed to believe that all would be okay. This had to be our little Christmas baby.

I started thinking about all the weddings we planned to attend over the next year. For some, I would be pregnant. For others, I would have to miss the wedding because I would have a newborn baby. Christmas would be spent close to home because I would be giving birth, and it would be the best Christmas ever.

In the few days following that ultrasound, I experienced some intense abdominal pain. I had been given progesterone suppositories to support the pregnancy, but those came with some not-so-fun side effects.

One morning, I reached for a bowl in the cabinet, and I doubled over in pain. I had been dealing with some significant constipation, and up until that moment, I had chalked my pain up to that. I had even called the doctor that morning to see if there was something he could recommend to get things "moving." All of which I tried. He had said if the pain continued or worsened, I should head to the emergency room.

When I couldn't even reach for a bowl without screaming out in pain, I knew things were bad. I leaned over the counter and reached for my phone to call Reid. "I need you to come home and take me to the ER. I am in a lot of pain, and I'm not sure what's going on."

"Okay, I'll be right there," he replied.

As I sat on our couch waiting for him, doubled over in pain, I realized I needed to go quicker. I got in the car and drove to the ER, praying I could make it there safely. Tears ran down my face as I went through the registration process and told them I was seven weeks pregnant. *God, please don't let this affect my pregnancy*, I prayed silently. I sat in the intake room, terrified and shivering.

Reid arrived shortly after, and they took us back to an exam room so the ER team could assess me. A few minutes after I sat down in the exam room, they brought a wheelchair and took me to another room to perform an ultrasound. The tech inserted the ultrasound wand, and I could tell by her silence that something was wrong.

After the ultrasound, they wheeled me back to the exam room, and the nurse hooked me up to various monitors.

Then, an ER doctor walked in.

Her eyes were full of sympathy as she said, "Unfortunately, your pregnancy is ectopic." My heart felt as if it was violently ripped out of my body, and I immediately started sobbing. I gasped for breath, and my body wretched forward as the monitors began beeping so loudly that I couldn't hear anything else. Two nurses came running in; the alarms had alerted the nurses' station I may be having a heart attack.

In the chaos and panic, I looked over at my husband and realized he had no clue what ectopic meant, and he was panicking, watching my reaction to the news. I gasped for air and told the ER doctor, "Tell him! Please explain... he doesn't know!"

As I regained my composure and assured the staff that I was not having a heart attack, just a panic attack, the doctor explained to my husband that the embryo was stuck in my fallopian tube. As a result, my left tube had ruptured, and I was bleeding internally. They would need to rush me into surgery, or this could be fatal. My OB-GYN was on his way to the hospital to perform the surgery. Once in surgery, my doctor would assess how much damage had been done and whether they would need to remove any of my reproductive organs.

Just as we were absorbing the news, a new team of medical professionals walked into the room. They handed Reid some paperwork to sign and explained that they were taking me to the operating room. Time was of the essence.

As they wheeled my hospital bed out of the room, I turned and asked Reid to call our family and a few friends. I did not want him sitting in the waiting room alone. He kissed me on the forehead and assured me he would, and then the nurse directed him towards the waiting room. She told him they would come and update him when the surgery was complete.

When the anesthesia began to wear off from my surgery, I realized that Reid, my parents, my sister, and my best friend were there in the post-op room. Their eyes were full of worry and pain. I could tell by my mom's face that if she could take away the intense pain I was feeling, she would. Not only did my parents lose a future grandchild, they almost lost their daughter as well.

The doctor entered the room and looked around at the room full of visitors. He asked if it was okay to provide an update now or if we needed some privacy. I asked that he share any information now… there was nothing we would hide from those standing in this room.

He explained he had removed my left fallopian tube, which contained our first baby. I was no longer pregnant, but the "good news" is that he only had to take out one fallopian tube. All my other reproductive organs were intact. I would need to let my body heal for a few months, but we could discuss more at his office during my follow-up visit.

For now, I needed to rest and take care of myself.

# Chapter 4

## The Aftermath

### Summer 2015 – Early 2016

The pain and trauma of that day in the ER *still* weigh heavily on me.

It was the most challenging day of my life up to that point. I felt I had done something wrong and failed everyone around me. Not only was I in physical and emotional pain as I recovered, but I watched those around me suffer.

Reid often came home from work to find me on the couch, cuddled up with Wrigley, mindlessly watching TV and avoiding eye contact. Since I worked from home, sometimes he wondered whether I had gotten any work done that day.

We had chosen to share our news with those closest to us, and now I felt the extra weight of their pain. I tried to hide my pain from others without much success.

The following several months were hard. I have always been the person who helps others. I didn't like this role reversal, where others constantly checked on me. I pretended as best I could that the loss wasn't affecting me because maybe then it wouldn't affect those around me as much. I carried on while my mind and emotions were in an unhealthy place.

I didn't feel I would ever be the person I was before. When I would share what happened with others, some would say, "At least you know you can get pregnant now." When it comes to losing a pregnancy, there is no "at least…"

One night, my best friend Denise and I went out for dinner. I had been forcing myself to do the things I usually loved, hoping it would help me get out of my dark place. The waitress became friendly with us as we sat there enjoying our dinner. Then she asked the dreaded question (I'm begging you, dear reader, never to ask a stranger this question): "Do you have kids?" I looked at Denise, and tears welled up in my eyes.

My entire body tensed as I said, "No, I don't."

She did not read the situation or assess my body language, so she continued to pry. "Do you plan to have kids?" she inquired.

I responded, "Yes, but I just had a pregnancy loss."

She then went on to tell me about her sister-in-law's cousin's friend who had a pregnancy loss and then had a healthy baby right after. She followed that statement with: "At least now you know you can get pregnant." I felt my face flush, and my palms became sweaty. I wanted to scream.

I know people mean well when they tell you about a friend of a friend (or even someone close to them) who suffered losses and went on to have healthy children. I realize they are trying to provide hope, but let me tell you what it did for me and many others I know who have dealt with the same situation. It negated the baby that I had carried. It made me feel as if my baby was insignificant and merely a stepping stone to the earthside baby I would hopefully have one day.

That baby was in my body, and I looked forward to all the moments I would have with them. And in a single moment, it had all been ripped away. Yes, I hoped to be pregnant again. But that next baby would not replace the one I had just lost. It would not erase the trauma of that day and make me wonder *what if* any less. The only response I needed was, "I'm sorry for your loss."

I desperately wanted her to quit prying into my personal life and let us enjoy our dinner.

Pregnancy and infertility can be challenging to talk about. No one knows what to say, and often, they say something hurtful without realizing it. I'm confident I've done the same to others in the past unintentionally.

Reid and I were advised to give my body a few months to heal after my surgery, and then we were back to trying. But this time, I was serious about it. I did *all* the things: I tracked my ovulation, I charted my basal body temperature, I did fertility yoga, I ate the things that claim to help with fertility, and I laid with my legs up after doing the deed. Getting pregnant and staying pregnant became my sole focus or, should I say, obsession. Sex was no longer sexy or spontaneous. It now became a scheduled activity based on my ovulation window.

During this time, we attended seven weddings. Two of my closest friends announced pregnancies. As they shared their news with me, I worked hard to put on my best happy face and congratulate them. Then I drove home bawling.

I felt like a terrible person. I should have been happy for my friends, and part of me was happy, but internally, I would throw a huge pity party for myself. Almost every event we attended ended with me in tears. It should have been a joyous time as so many friends started their married lives and began growing their families. But it felt like I had a massive rain cloud over my head, and it could release a torrential downpour any minute.

Meeting friends for dinner filled me with anxiety because I convinced myself they would be announcing a pregnancy. As everyone ordered their drinks at the restaurant, I would listen carefully to who didn't order alcohol, and if any of the girls didn't, my internal spiral would continue. I never believed the "I don't feel like drinking tonight" or "I'm on antibiotics" comments and assumed that meant they were pregnant. God forbid someone decides not to drink when out for dinner.

The constant stories of people having pregnancy losses and then going on to have healthy children shortly after convinced me that it would happen to us, too. But it didn't. At least not when and how I wanted.

My social media newsfeed overflowed with pregnancy announcements and newborn babies. These posts had always brought me joy and hope, but now reading them left me feeling heartbroken, filled with jealousy and rage.

Every wedding we attended had at least one person with a pregnant belly, and I did my best to avoid that person at all costs. At one wedding, we were chatting in a circle of friends, and one guy told us he just "looked at his wife, and she became pregnant." He then joked that he didn't understand how we couldn't "just make it happen." Cue the massive breakdown and another night ending in tears.

After leaving another wedding, I called my mom at midnight in a full-on panic attack. Watching other families dance with their kids, and then a friend with a pregnant belly dance with her husband had set me off. I sobbed into the phone and pleaded with her to tell me this pain would lessen. My grief for the baby we had just lost consumed my every fiber, and I feared I would never get to hold a child in my arms. My mom tried her best to help mend my broken heart, as she always did.

I had another close friend who had recently had a miscarriage, but she was "fine." Why wasn't I fine? She was also now pregnant again.

Have you ever been told by your doctor to avoid certain foods, and then it seems those foods are constantly in front of you? That's how I felt: everywhere I looked, there were pregnancies.

In every show or movie we watched, someone ended up pregnant. I would always feel it coming. The ache would creep into my body as the storyline shifted. I can't tell you how many times Reid and I switched TV series entirely because a pregnancy storyline had been added.

Every time we went to eat at a restaurant, they sat us next to a pregnant woman or a family with an adorable baby. At least, that is how it felt. My immense pain wouldn't even allow me to look at the baby.

Each month, when I started my period, I had a major meltdown. That single pink line on the pregnancy test felt like a failure to do something that came so easily to many others. For days after, I would be consumed with anger.

I used to believe everything happened for a reason and that life would work out as it should. Now, anger seemed to be the only emotion I felt. Don't dare tell me about God's plan. I didn't want to hear anything about a plan that meant so much pain. How could hurt and sadness be part of some ultimate plan, and if it was, how badly had I screwed up in the past to deserve this? I had made my fair share of mistakes but felt I was a decent and compassionate human, so it made no sense why I would be punished.

While my emotions were still in a whirlwind from our incredible loss, Reid's health had started to decline. It was slow at first. He would come home from work every day and nap on the couch. He also began experiencing constant itching, like a deep internal itch that no amount of scratching would alleviate. He went in for regular colonoscopies (to check on the UC) and ERCPs (endoscopic procedures to check on the PSC), which started showing more scarring and blockages in his bile ducts. His liver numbers were also slowly deteriorating.

The doctors gave him medications to attempt to reduce the itching, but those came with even worse side effects. Reid's weight kept dropping despite eating a regular diet. He kept experiencing intense pains in his stomach from his ulcerative colitis, which would sometimes leave him in the fetal position until they went away.

We were concerned about his health, but his medical team told us there wasn't much we could do at that point other than what we were doing. Therefore, we put most of our energy into trying to create a family.

We were no longer a fun couple to be around. Our health challenges felt all-consuming, and we struggled to carry on normal conversations with others. Therefore, we limited our interactions and disconnected ourselves from those around us.

We still attended the weddings and showers we had committed to, but every conversation would inevitably turn toward our struggles, and we'd always duck out early. Either Reid wasn't feeling great, or I was holding back tears because someone asked when we'd be having children or inadvertently brought up the fact that we were still childless while everyone else around us seemed to have no issues in that department.

So much for that marital bliss everyone talks about.

As Christmas of 2015 approached, I became even more anxious. We should have been getting ready for our baby. I usually love the holidays; Thanksgiving and Christmas are my favorites. That year, I lived in a shell of the person I used to be. I dreaded the many family parties we had scheduled.

Reid's sister, Sarah, gave birth to a son in September of that year. She and her family, along with Reid's parents, drove to Houston that Christmas to spend the holiday at our house. Reid's aunt also flew in for the first Christmas with the new baby. I was so happy to have our first nephew with us, but I couldn't help but look at him and wonder why we couldn't also be celebrating with *our* first baby.

I vividly remember all my emotions that Christmas Day—our baby's due date. I can even remember where I sat on the couch as we opened presents while I choked back tears. My nephew was being passed around as we all took turns opening presents, but I avoided holding him. I just couldn't.

We had all bought gifts for him and took turns opening them, oohing and aahing over the baby clothes, books, and toys. I had vowed I would not make this about me, so I became determined not to let anyone see how I felt inside. I took deep breaths several times to keep myself from having the breakdown I felt bubbling up to the surface. I made it through all the gift-giving, then got up and walked into our bedroom. I barely shut the door to our room before I started crying.

Why did we have to feel this pain? Why wasn't our baby here with us? There is a 2% chance of a pregnancy being ectopic. Why did that slight chance happen to us? Would we *ever* have a baby, or would I always be the aunt? Would I ever be a worthy mother through the pain I felt?

Reid came in to check on me and didn't know what to say or do. Men seem to process these things differently, and Reid can compartmentalize. But he still felt it, and it hurt him to see me in so much pain. His family knew I was having a hard time, but I tried to hide it for the rest of their trip so I didn't take away from their joy.

In January of 2016, my pity party was in full swing. I remember telling Denise, "Something's got to give. I don't think I can take one more thing."

As I drove to work the following week, I picked up the phone to call my grandma, as I did at least once a week. My phone rang while in my hand…my dad was calling. He said, "Mema passed out, and they told me to come now. I don't know what's happening, but the ambulance is on the way." My Grandpa was in poor health, fighting lymphoma, and Mema had been taking care of him. She had been our family's glue and seemed relatively healthy.

That day, my aunt and uncle found her on the floor of their living room and started performing CPR, but she never took another breath. The unexpected death of my Mema shook me to my core.

At that point, I realized I was so sad that a healthy baby and a healthy husband wouldn't make me feel better. I had been chasing this dream of a happy, healthy family and had lost myself in the process. I had to get help, work on myself, and stop pretending to be okay.

I found a local therapist and started going in for regular appointments with her. It helped to talk to this sweet older lady. In some regards, it felt like I was talking to my grandma.

I started opening up more to those around me, sharing my true feelings, and leaning on our support system. If people don't realize how badly you are hurting and you don't allow them in, they can't support you. I started talking about what happened and how it made me feel: resentful, heartbroken, and defeated.

I even shared all those feelings, like jealousy, that I felt terrible for having. And the support came flooding in. It made a world of difference. Did it help me get pregnant? No, of course not. But it helped me realize how deep my depression had gone, and getting pregnant wasn't going to solve my problems.

I started focusing on making myself a whole person again. I began praying again (remember, I was pretty mad at God), I deleted Facebook and Instagram from my phone, and had Denise change my password (fewer pregnancy announcements if you're off social media.) I focused on doing things that made me happy. I had to be even more selfish for a little while to return to a point where I could be normal.

My outlook slowly started to improve.

# Chapter 5

## A Turn for the Better?

### 2016

In January of 2016, the same month my Mema passed away, I went in for my annual woman's visit. It was the first time I visited my OB-GYN office after our check-up from the ectopic pregnancy.

That visit was so much more difficult than I thought it would be. My little sister, Megan, was with me as I sat in the waiting room. I looked around at the other women with their pregnant bellies, and my hands started to sweat. I felt a massive rock in my stomach, and my breath quickened. I looked at Megan and whispered, "I don't know if I can be here right now. I didn't realize it would hit me like this."

They called me back to the exam room before I could plan my escape. Megan offered to go with me, but I nervously shook my head and assured her I would be okay.

Once I was in the room, I climbed onto the exam table. Before the nurse even started talking, I burst into tears. She looked at me with pity and apologized for what I was going through. The doctor came in shortly after to see the tears still streaming down my face. In a compassionate voice, he offered his condolences. "We would really like a referral to a fertility specialist. I know that's where we will end up," I pleaded.

He replied that he could not refer us until we'd been trying for a year after the ectopic pregnancy. I mentally marked my calendar for June.

I spent the next few months trying not to obsess over the fact that I now had a deadline. Either we would get pregnant, or we'd start seeing a fertility specialist.

These potential outcomes left me with mixed feelings. I felt a glimmer of hope that we'd have more options with a specialist, but we were also admitting we needed help to get pregnant. Isn't that supposed to be something special between husband and wife? Not for us, I guess.

In June 2016, we had our first appointment with a Reproductive Endocrinologist (a fertility specialist). We sat nervously in the fertility clinic's waiting room as we waited for them to call my name. I glanced around at the other couples sitting there and wondered how far along they were in this process. *Are they as nervous as I am right now?* I thought. The radio in the corner of the room buzzed a staticky local station. I wanted so badly to fix the radio. But I sat frozen in my seat.

The nurse called my name and took us back to Dr. Griffith's office. He immediately put me at ease as he greeted us at the door with a warm smile and a firm handshake. He invited us to sit in the chairs facing his desk. He had a laid-back demeanor, and he didn't skirt around the fact that no one wanted to be in a position to need his services.

We explained our current situation and shared Reid's chronic illnesses with Dr. Griffith. He suggested we start by testing Reid to see if his health issues were affecting his fertility. A week after our initial meeting, we learned Reid was perfectly fine (in the fertility department, at least) and that we needed to order additional testing to figure out where the issue lay with me.

When my bloodwork results returned two weeks later, Dr. Griffith shared that my AMH (anti-müllerian hormone) level was 0.5. I was 30 years old, but this test indicated I had the egg count of a 45-year-old (that is my paraphrasing, obviously not the medical definition.) *Fabulous.*

He broke down our options and showed us all the charts. This doctor's approach included honest direction but also compassion for his patients.

He sat and talked with us as long as needed and answered all of Reid's statistical and analytical questions. He told us we could try doing an IUI (Intrauterine insemination), but time was of the essence with my AMH being so low. He suggested we move straight to IVF (In vitro fertilization), as our chances were better with that process.

Dr. Griffith warned us that IVF was not a guarantee to get pregnant, so he couldn't promise it would work for us. There is a 60-65% chance of IVF being successful, so it was possible we would have to go through multiple rounds before we would have a baby in our arms.

At that time, needles terrified me, and I would panic days before I had bloodwork or a shot. Somehow, I knew I would have to push past it—my desire to have children had to be greater than that fear.

I asked the doctor what I/we could do to improve our chances of IVF success. He gave me a list of supplements and suggested I see an acupuncturist specializing in fertility. Finally, someone provided hope and an action plan. Sure, there was still a chance it wouldn't work, but this was our best shot (literally!). I assured him I would do every item on that list to better our chances.

He then walked us to the next office to talk with their financial counselor, Haley. She laid out all the costs for us. Each round of IVF would cost roughly $16,000-19,000 before medications, which could be an additional $2,000-8,000. She gave us a list of possible creditors and grants we could apply for, but most of the cost would need to be paid upfront.

Anyone who has said, "At least you can do IVF!" has obviously never sat down and had those conversations to determine what is involved in the process – mentally, physically, and financially.

I remembered a friend from high school who had shared on Facebook that she did IVF and now had a baby boy. Later that day, I contacted her, and she talked me through the process. I always like to know what I'm getting into and will use all available resources.

I will never forget that during that conversation, she said, "We were very lucky; it worked on the first round for us." They were *lucky* because most of the people she knew who had gone through the process did not have a baby after one round of IVF. The doctor had just spelled out our chances, but I still thought we'd go through one round and have a baby in our arms. Hearing her say that was a bit of a reality check.

The fertility clinic sent me a 20-page document explaining the IVF process in full. They also sent a breakdown of all the costs. I read and re-read all of that and then sent it to my boss, Julie. She and I were very close, and I wanted her to know what to expect as we went through the process. This would affect my job, as I would need to go in regularly for monitoring. I also anticipated being a complete mess (even more so than I had been) as I would be pumped full of hormones. Julie always supported me and was ready to take this on with us.

Reid and I started crunching numbers to determine whether we could begin the process immediately. He is a mechanical engineer for an oil and gas company, and I was a project manager for a relocation company. We both had well-paying jobs but did not have $19,000+ just lying around to hand over. We called a credit union in my hometown and secured a loan. I was planning to drive to Huntsville to get the check (and give the loan officer a big hug, as she had worked hard to get us a loan quickly) the following week.

Based on when my cycle should start, we were set to begin the process on July 22nd. We had already planned a trip to Chicago the weekend prior, so we decided to live it up before starting this challenging process. We spent a few great days exploring one of Reid's favorite cities. Of course, we caught a Cubs game there, so I got to live the Cubs fan experience in person.

I came back completely relaxed and ready to start IVF.

On July 21st, 2016, I woke up and felt a little flu-like. I decided to take a pregnancy test but didn't expect anything from it. I jumped in the shower, started getting dressed, and remembered I'd left the test in the bathroom and hadn't checked it. To my surprise, there was a double line again. I couldn't believe it.

It had been 15 months since our last positive, and I fully expected I would not be able to get pregnant without IVF. I mean, we were going in to meet with the doctor the next day to start our first round of IVF.

This had to be a total God thing. I stood in the bathroom holding the test as chills covered my body.

In shock, I made an appointment with Dr. Griffith. They confirmed the double lines were correct, and I was pregnant again, but my progesterone and estrogen were low. They prescribed hormones for me to start taking immediately. This wasn't abnormal, as some women have to take supplemental hormones throughout their entire pregnancy.

We once again shared the news quickly with a few of our closest friends and immediate family. While it hurt to feel their pain the last time, I had come to realize that I would need them for whatever lay ahead. Also, as I've mentioned, I'm not good at keeping secrets.

Everyone agreed this was meant to be. I got pregnant the day before we were supposed to start our first round of IVF. That was a sign we didn't need medical intervention. As scared as I felt, I held onto the hope that this could be our earth-side baby. We had some hurdles to jump, but we now had a fertility doctor closely monitoring me, so I was hopeful we had the resources we needed to support this pregnancy.

I mentioned that most women have a 2% chance of their pregnancy being ectopic. Now that I had only one tube and had experienced one ectopic pregnancy, they told me my chances had jumped to 20%. Knowing this, we were pretty anxious about that first ultrasound. I had bloodwork every 2-3 days for the first week or two. The numbers were rising, but my progesterone and estrogen remained lower than normal. This didn't seem super alarming, so we continued to hold onto hope.

We had our first ultrasound and saw the embryo in the uterus. Thankfully, we had avoided another ectopic pregnancy. Several days later, we saw the heartbeat. The baby was measuring a little behind, but since this pregnancy was spontaneous, we were assured it could be a matter of dates being off a bit.

I continued to go to the fertility clinic multiple times a week and had one to two ultrasounds a week. Reid accompanied me for each of the ultrasounds, and together, we watched the baby grow. As we passed each milestone, our excitement grew.

At this point, we had told all our immediate family and closest friends. Between nine and ten weeks, we figured we were in the clear to share our news with our extended family. The pregnancy was far enough along that the chances of miscarriage had dropped to five percent.

I downloaded an app that shows the baby's daily development. Our baby was the size of a grape, had all his/her essential body parts, including eyes, and was starting to grow teeth.

During Labor Day weekend, we had a get-together with one side of my extended family at our house (someone had already spilled the beans on the other side of the family.) My mom, sister, and I had planned to surprise them with the news. We love to play games, and one of the games we would play is similar to charades, where you each get a few slips of paper. You write down anything you'd like on each slip of paper, and they all go into one bowl together. We'd take turns going up in front of the group and drawing one of the slips of paper. You'd have to get the others to guess what it said. I had put one in, saying, "Reid and Abby are having a baby!"

My mom, sister, Reid, and I all anxiously awaited as each paper was drawn, wondering if it would be the one. We wanted to make sure to get that moment on video.

Finally, after drawing what felt like every paper in the bowl, it was my mom's turn. She got up in front of us, opened her slip of paper, and gave Megan and me a knowing look. She started acting it out, and my sister couldn't take it any longer; she just screamed out, "REID AND ABBY ARE HAVING A BABY!!!" Everyone laughed a bit at first and then realized what was happening. My cousin jumped up in realization, and everyone came in for hugs. This would be the first baby of all the cousins and my maternal grandma's first great-grandchild. We were all so excited; I don't remember if we finished the game.

I then sent the video out to anyone else who didn't know. Our dreams were coming true, and we were *finally* having a baby. I signed up for a baby registry online and started searching for cribs. I had a strong feeling I was carrying a boy, so I started a Pinterest board dedicated to nursery décor for boys. I ordered onesies and maternity clothes. Things were finally happening. Our time to become parents had at last arrived.

# Chapter 6

# It All Comes Crashing Down

## Fall 2016

Two days after we shared the news with our family at our Labor Day party, I had another ultrasound. We had at least one a week for the last five weeks, so we knew what to expect. Reid had a big meeting at work, so I told him not to worry about going. It would be the usual: we'd see the baby, and I would do more bloodwork.

I arrived at the appointment feeling pretty chipper. I greeted the phlebotomist, whom I knew well by now. She knew which vein in which arm was best to use, as I had some that were harder to draw from than others. My nurse stood next to me during the blood draw. "How are you feeling?" she asked with a smile.

I told her more nausea was setting in, so hopefully, that meant the baby was growing well. After the bloodwork, they took me back to an exam room. I undressed from the waist down and sat on the exam table with the modesty sheet draped over my bottom half. Dr. Griffith came in with one of the nurses. We chatted, and the nurse began the ultrasound.

She measured the baby, and the reading came up at eight weeks and three days. Wait a second; that's what it said last week.

Dr. Griffith stood over her shoulder and studied the monitor on the ultrasound machine. He turned the monitor towards him, asked the nurse to let him try, and grabbed the wand they used for the transvaginal ultrasound.

He inserted the wand again, and then he got quiet.

He put his hand on the front of my shin and, in a soft voice, said, "Abby…"

My heart sank, and I immediately pleaded, "Please don't say it."

He responded, "I'm so sorry, Abby, but there's no longer a heartbeat."

I am confident my sobs could be heard in the waiting room as I gasped for breath, feeling like my heart had just been ripped from my chest once again.

*How could this happen? How could we be getting this kind of news again? Why did my perfect baby with a heartbeat of 174 suddenly die?* The doctor explained that this was considered a missed miscarriage, which meant the baby was no longer alive, but my body had not recognized that fact.

He asked me to get dressed and join him in his office to talk more. Once in his office, we called Reid on speakerphone. He stepped out of his meeting, expecting to hear good news. I said, "I need you to get to someplace private where you can talk."

The doctor explained to Reid that we had lost the baby. At this point, he really wasn't sure why this happened. I could hear Reid's sniffles through the phone as he absorbed the news.

Dr. Griffith said we were far enough along that he didn't want me to pass the baby naturally. He recommended a D&C (dilation and curettage procedure) to remove the baby from my uterus. In doing that, we could also run tests on the tissue to determine what happened. Talking about my baby in medical terms and calling it "tissue" still makes my skin crawl, but that was the reality of the situation.

My whole body ached as we talked, and I kept my hands folded over my abdomen.

I wanted to schedule the procedure immediately. I had already been carrying a baby who was no longer alive for a week, and I didn't even know it. I did not want this to go on longer than it had to. Dr. Griffith picked up the phone to call the surgery center and scheduled the D&C for the following day.

Dr. Griffith was so caring. I don't know how long I sat in his office crying. When I finally got up to leave, he hugged me and asked if I'd like to slip out the back door.

I walked quickly to my car, avoiding eye contact with anyone on the way there. Once I turned on the ignition, the sobs came even more violently.

After a few minutes and several deep breaths, I collected myself enough to call my mom. She was used to the weekly updates by this point, so she cheerily answered the phone. "How's our baby?" she sang into the phone. I could feel her smile on the other end as she waited for an update on her grandbaby.

I burst into tears again and said, "There's no more heartbeat. Our baby died." Those were difficult words to say. Judging by her response, they were just as challenging to hear. I have never heard my mom cry the way she did that day.

Once we both calmed down, she said she would head to our house soon. I sat in the hospital parking lot and called my dad and Denise. Then I called Julie so she could cover my meetings the next day. I had already told four people (five, including Reid) that our baby had died, and I couldn't do it anymore. I asked the people I had already told to spread the word.

I could not believe we were here. We had seen our baby and had heard the heartbeat multiple times. I even picked out a crib. *Was this really happening??*

I now had a new worst day of my life.

Reid came home from work shortly after, and we both had a good, ugly cry. We were in disbelief, and our hearts were broken. Things had been going so well. We got pregnant **the day before** we were supposed to start IVF, so we thought God was sending us a signal, but it wasn't the one we had hoped and prayed for.

Throughout the day, I went from crying hysterically to staring at the TV in a daze and back again. Denise sat on one side of me, holding my hand, as my mom was on the other, stroking my hair. My sister sat next to my mom, and I could feel her wanting to do anything to make this better for us.

I had finally reached the point where I felt relaxed about the pregnancy, allowed myself to be happy, and looked forward to the future.

All of it got ripped away with one phrase: "There's no heartbeat." I do not wish that moment on my worst enemy.

Neither Reid nor I knew what to do, so we appreciated having people around to take care of us. They ensured we ate, and Denise called my OB-GYN to cancel my next appointment. We had been at the point in the pregnancy where you graduate from the fertility doctor to your regular OB-GYN, which is a big deal. I had our first appointment set up for the following week. I didn't have it in me to call and cancel.

While the three of them were there, they also went around our house and collected all the baby items I had bought or had been gifted to put away. That included books, onesies, stuffed animals, pregnancy journals, ultrasound pictures, etc. I just wanted everything stuffed in a box out of my sight.

The following day, we went in for the D&C.

As we walked into the surgery center's waiting room, our parents greeted us with somber faces. I barely spoke, and I gave each of them a hug. Reid went to the reception desk to let them know we had arrived. I looked around at the décor of the waiting room, which they had attempted to make bright and airy, but I felt as though I had darkness all around me.

I couldn't believe we were going through this awful reality. Dr. Griffith came in to talk to us before the procedure, and we had our list of questions: What would this mean for our future fertility? What does he think happened? Could I have caused this to happen somehow? When would we get the results? What are the chances of this happening again?

He had answers to some, and some he didn't. He was patient while we went through our list and addressed each question as best he could.

After speaking with the doctor, a nurse came to walk me back to the operating room. I walked into the cold, sterile room, and immediately, my body began to tremble. I climbed onto the table, and after I laid down, an anesthesiologist put an oxygen mask over my face. Tears streamed down my face as I fell asleep.

The procedure didn't take long (at least for me; it may have been much longer in the waiting room.) I woke up feeling so empty and cramping. I wanted to be anywhere but there at that moment, and my heart felt shattered into pieces. They gave me morphine since I asked to "not feel anything for the rest of the day – physically or emotionally."

The nurse wheeled me into the elevator as Reid had gone to pull the car up. My mother-in-law was in the elevator with me, and I remember feeling like a shell of a person sitting in that wheelchair. I stared straight ahead and didn't speak a word. I could sense her sorrowful gaze on me, but I couldn't bring myself to meet her eyes. She clutched her sweater in her arms as pain and sadness filled the elevator.

I had a work project that weekend, which was good since I wanted to distract myself as much as possible. I needed to accept where we were and that the future we had been planning was no longer a reality.

With our first loss, I was scheduled to oversee a substantial 400-person relocation the next day at work. Naturally, I had to hand that one over. The day my grandma suddenly passed away, I had just started a residential relocation project and had to turn that one over to a co-worker. It now seemed I had a pattern I needed to break.

The day after my D&C, I oversaw a relocation for a company I used to work for. I did not want to miss it since many of my friends still worked there, and I had close ties with the company. Mentally, I just needed to accomplish something. I needed to feel I had some control over something in my life.

My boss and co-workers were wonderful. They knew I wouldn't be 100% for the project, but I felt I needed to be there. The team filled in all the gaps.

I was still experiencing some pain from the procedure, so I could not be as involved as I had hoped (and I quickly learned it's not a good idea to be on your feet for several hours after taking major painkillers.) The move went well, thanks mainly to my co-workers and boss. It felt good to change the pattern a bit and have a small win.

A couple of days later, Julie called me. After inquiring how I was doing, she insisted, "I want you to take two weeks off with pay." She knew I had been avoiding dealing with the loss, and she saw first-hand how much the last one affected me.

At first, I argued. "I'm okay; I need to stay focused on work right now."

"I am not asking; I'm telling you. You need to take some time off. I'm worried about you," she pushed.

I reluctantly agreed. What was I going to do for two weeks? I certainly did not want to sit around and feel sorry for myself. I thought about things I would enjoy doing, and I planned to do them.

I went shopping with my mother-in-law to decorate their new home. They had recently moved to Houston because Reid's health worried them to the point where they wanted to be closer. I redecorated parts of our home and had lunches and mani/pedis with friends.

I entered a phase where I wanted everything to be different, so I colored my hair red—like—RED. Reid grew a beard - that had more to do with the Cubs being in the playoffs, but still, it was a change I welcomed with open arms. I bought a new couch (I wanted a new house, but Reid thought that was a bit much.) I did everything I could not to return to where I had been the previous year.

The day after my D&C, I went to see the counselor I had seen earlier that year but realized I needed something a little different this time. My mom's best friend found a therapist who specializes in infertility and pregnancy loss.

I began seeing Jules, the new therapist, the week after we lost our second baby. It made a world of difference. She talked with couples who had faced the same issues we were dealing with daily, so she knew the best way to help work through those feelings. She also ran a support group once a month and invited me and Reid to attend, which we happily accepted.

I had been through this once and tried to conquer it without asking for help. I knew that wasn't the way to go, so if people offered help, I accepted.

During the following weeks, I tried to allow myself to be sad and not tuck it away when those feelings came creeping in. But I refused to get stuck there. I would have my cry (sometimes I would "schedule" it for later if it wasn't a good time – great suggestion from my therapist,) and then I would get up and do something. Sometimes, I practiced gratitude and added to my list of things I was grateful for. The silver lining of going through tough times was realizing how much support we had. And I truly felt it.

Exactly three weeks after our loss, we went to the fertility doctor to read the results of the products of conception (POC) test they performed to try to learn why our baby's heart had stopped. Reid and I talked before the appointment, and I said I wanted to know the sex of the baby. He didn't. He said for him, it would change it from "losing a baby" to "losing a son or daughter," and it would be even harder to process. After some discussion, we agreed not to find out.

We sat in Dr. Griffith's office, and he turned his computer monitor to show us our results. Right there, in the middle, it said, "MALE." My heart sank (not my doctor's fault; we should have said that upfront.)

He explained that the baby had triploid syndrome (also called triploidy), which meant the baby had three of each chromosome. Most babies with triploidy miscarry, but the few who do make it to birth only live a few days. The good news - if you can call it that - is that it was typically not a recurring problem, and nothing we could have done would have changed the outcome.

Of course, we asked the doctor, "Where do we go from here?"

"What do you feel is best?" he countered.

I felt that getting pregnant the day before we were to start IVF showed we could get pregnant on our own again, and I wasn't ready for IVF. We all agreed that Reid and I would try to conceive naturally for six months. The doctor wanted us to come back and discuss IVF again if we weren't pregnant by then. Another deadline. He also mentioned that my hCG, the primary pregnancy hormone, needed to get back to zero before we were able to try again. That meant more bloodwork to watch that number trend down.

After we left the clinic, I did more research on triploidy babies and learned that it occurs in 1-3% of confirmed pregnancies. If you haven't figured it out by now, we tend to hit all the small odds. I also learned that 2/3 of triploidy pregnancies are lost in the first trimester, and the other third are lost later in the pregnancy or after birth. Ultimately, the child cannot survive with three sets of chromosomes. I realized then it had been a blessing we lost the baby when we did. I know that sounds terrible, but I believe it would have been even harder if it happened later in the pregnancy. It helped me to have answers and know what happened.

For the next three (long) months, I went to the doctor every week for more bloodwork. Each time I pulled into the hospital parking lot, it reminded me of that dreadful day I sat there calling our people to tell them our baby's heart had stopped beating. I refused to park on the same side of the parking lot, even if that meant circling the lot a few times and waiting for another car to leave.

While my body was no longer carrying a baby, I still had the pregnancy hormones in my system, and they were taking their time going down. That was one of the hardest things to process. I no longer carried a baby, but at times, I still felt pregnant. My hCG went down so slowly that it took 12 weeks before we were back at zero. Not being able to get a start on our next deadline frustrated me, but we were strictly advised not to. I also experienced hair loss, like many moms do postpartum.

One day, a close friend who had become pregnant during those tough months for us brought her newborn over. She and I sat on the couch, and I held her baby. During the conversation, she removed her hat and showed me her postpartum hair loss. As calmly as possible, I looked at her and said, "Jess, I am also losing my hair. But I don't have a baby to show for it." She had always been so sensitive to what we were going through and had no idea how her complaint would hit me. Fortunately, she was a friend I could be honest with. She apologized, and I knew she truly didn't realize how insensitive her complaint was. It was a valid complaint; it was just said to the wrong person at the wrong time.

# Chapter 7

## Cautiously Optimistic

### Winter 2016–Spring 2017

On December 1st, 2016, Dr. Griffith finally cleared us to stop avoiding conception. Here we go again.

I finally realized I had no control over the process and that I couldn't revolve my life around trying to get pregnant. No matter how hard others tried to convince me, I had to come to that realization on my own.

Reid and I both decided we weren't going to *try*, but we weren't going to *not try*. I was done doing ovulation tests and charting my basal body temperature. We wanted to enjoy our lives, and all we could do was hope things worked out as they should. I had spent the last two and a half years planning my life around hoping to become pregnant or being pregnant. I could not live in that mindset any longer.

I continued seeing the acupuncturist Dr. Griffith had recommended, which reduced my anxiety and made me feel like I was still doing something to help the process. I had seen the difference in my overall physical and emotional well-being. They worked with me to manage my stress, focus on egg quality, and improve my health and fertility. I had once been a girl who was terrified of needles, but now, I would willingly lay there with tiny needles all over my body each week.

Now that we were trying/not trying to get pregnant, Chris, my acupuncturist, recommended I go on a low-carb diet. He had read studies that showed a correlation between low AMH levels and inflammation in the gut. As much as I loved my carbs, I vowed to do it. Two years into trying for a baby, and all we had to show for it was two pregnancy losses… I could handle a simple diet change.

Over the Christmas holiday, I had all sorts of pregnancy symptoms. I assumed they were in my head, as usual. You may remember that December 25th was our first due date, so I thought it was just wishful thinking to help me overcome a difficult time. No way would we be one of those couples who got pregnant the first month (of trying again).

On January 2nd, 2017, I felt off again. I took a test and then got back in bed. Reid got up to use the bathroom shortly after and said, "Your pregnancy test is negative. Maybe you're getting sick." Probably.

I went into the bathroom a bit later and squinted at the test. There it was—a faint line. It wasn't glaringly obvious, so Reid didn't notice it, but it was there. I told Reid, "There is a line. But it's super faint." We didn't celebrate. I'm not sure we even smiled. We knew a faint line at this point in my cycle probably meant another miscarriage.

I called Dr. Griffith's office and scheduled an appointment for later that day. Anxiety set in, and my nervous system went into overdrive.

On the way to the doctor, I called my mom and said, "I'm pregnant, BUT I don't know anything yet. The line is faint, so my numbers are low, and we're not celebrating yet." Thankfully, my mom didn't throw the usual excessive positivity my way. If I heard her declare once more that I **would** be a mom one day and "my time would come," I would snap at her (again).

I went in for bloodwork, and we tried to stay busy that afternoon while waiting for the results. We weren't expecting good news. Sure, we hoped for it, but we didn't expect it.

The nurse finally called me that afternoon, asked me the date of my last period, and shared that my hCG was at 26, which was low, but it was confirmation that we were pregnant. She asked if I still had progesterone suppositories and estrogen pills from the last pregnancy, which I did, so she directed me to start taking them. They scheduled me to come in for more bloodwork the next day and said we would need to see the numbers increasing before we knew more. We were still not celebrating.

We had more bloodwork over the next couple of weeks, which showed my numbers increasing, but not at a standard rate. We tried to remain cautiously optimistic and mostly avoided discussing the pregnancy. Here's the thing about being pregnant after multiple losses: we never felt like we could fully relax and celebrate the pregnancy. When you've had the kind of luck we had, you learn to expect the worst.

I didn't do anything that I had done the last time. I didn't download the apps that told me about the baby's daily development. I didn't write in a pregnancy journal, and I didn't text my closest family and friends each time I got the results of my bloodwork. I asked those who knew not to ask questions or check on me. I told them, "No news is good news," as I didn't want to feel their stress on top of mine. I tried to pretend I wasn't pregnant, so I didn't think about it all the time.

On January 17th, 2017, we went in for an ultrasound and confirmed the baby was in the uterus, so we dodged another ectopic pregnancy. At that point, the doctor thought everything looked okay; he just questioned how far along I was. When we got the bloodwork back later that day, all my numbers were low. While we began to worry, Dr. Griffith didn't want to call it quits on the baby just yet.

We increased the supplemental hormones and went in for more testing two days later. Things didn't change much.

The following Tuesday, we went to the fertility clinic for another ultrasound and bloodwork. The baby hadn't grown much since the week prior, and we still didn't see a heartbeat, so we were sure this wouldn't work out as we had hoped. Later that afternoon, I received a call from Dr. Griffith. He said, "I'm so sorry, but the baby is no longer viable. I hate to be giving you this kind of news again."

I understood this would probably be the outcome and had been preparing for it for weeks. I felt pretty numb as he told me once again that this would not be a baby we'd ever hold in our arms.

"So what do we do now?" I asked.

He gave me the option to come off the hormones and let my body miscarry naturally - which could take days or weeks - or I could go in for another D&C. I chose the latter. I knew the process of a D&C and knew we could also find out what happened that way. I felt that waiting for my body to miscarry naturally sounded like an agonizing process. Each day, I would be wondering if that was the day my body would expel the baby. We scheduled the procedure for two days later.

A couple of years ago, I worked with someone who had three miscarriages. I remember talking to her about helping me with a project. She shared that she was having another D&C but could be there the day after. I told her I didn't think it was a good idea, as she needed time to heal and process, but her response was, "I feel numb at this point. We've been through this a couple of times." I completely understood what she meant now. Yes, I was sad. But we'd been through this. I knew what to expect, what I'd need, and how I'd feel. Somehow, it got easier. Or maybe I had learned to compartmentalize better.

While I felt I was handling things better this time around, I would still have *those days*. You know, the days when you felt like you couldn't even get out of bed in the morning.

Pregnancy loss is grief, and grief comes in waves. With the loss, there are always reminders of what could have been. But I leaned on the support around me, and this time, I had more resources to help me get through those hard days.

A few weeks later, we heard from our nurse that our third baby, another boy, had trisomy 11 (the baby had three of the 11th chromosome instead of two). I was actually relieved it was a trisomy. How terrible is that? What I mean is that we had a common miscarriage, not one of these 2% chance events.

Later that week, we met with Dr. Griffith to discuss the loss. He explained that with Trisomy 11, the baby wouldn't have survived outside of the womb, and it's unlikely we would have even made it past eight weeks.

He explained that all three of our losses had been pretty random. There is no explanation as to why one person would have an ectopic, a triploidy, and a trisomy pregnancy. Although it may sound frustrating, it was a relief to us because it meant there probably wasn't an underlying issue with one of us (other than my low AMH).

He suggested that we do a miscarriage panel on me (which requires 17 vials of blood) and a chromosome test on Reid. He didn't think it was likely we'd find something else – in fact, he said there's a 3% chance that there's a more significant issue with one of us – but it wouldn't hurt to check so we could potentially avoid another heartbreak.

The tests would check for any genetic problems such as chromosomal abnormalities, inflammation, and any auto-immune issues that could be related to our infertility. Since we had done POC (products of conception) testing on the last two babies, he knew these losses weren't due to issues with one of us, but he hoped this would give us some peace of mind for future pregnancies.

Just like last time, we had to check to make sure my hCG level was back down to zero. Thank God it was.

Our story had changed significantly since we first met with Dr. Griffith. We went from trying for 15 months and being told we needed to do IVF to getting pregnant twice on our own. The last one, we had only been trying for one month. He felt comfortable continuing with our plan to try to conceive without IVF unless we weren't able to get pregnant again on our own in the next several months and as long as the genetic testing came back normal.

He said, "Whether you guys try on your own or I help you with medical intervention – ultimately, it's all up to God." We knew he was right, so we left it in His hands and prayed for the best!

We then went back into the mode of trying/not trying. We were hopeful it would happen, but I tried not to apply the extra stress and pressure. We wanted to focus on living our lives and enjoying this time as much as we could. We were now hopeful for our future and confident we'd have a baby at some point, in some way.

The day after my second D&C, I seriously considered starting a blog. I wrote the first post and shared it with Reid, explaining that I wanted to start writing about our journey to help process everything and let others know they're not alone.

Reid was more private, so I wasn't sure he would be on board with us putting it all out there in this way. We sat down that night to discuss the idea, and Reid said, "If it will help you, then I want you to do it." But he was concerned about people online being insensitive in their replies, either intentionally or by accident. "If it hurts more than it helps at any point, I want you to walk away from it."

I began writing, and all my feelings poured out through my fingers as I typed out our story. I put my raw emotions out there for the world to see, and in came a flood of support from others. The number of people who sent me private messages saying they, too, had experienced losses amazed me. I had others who reached out and said they had a friend or family member struggling with infertility and wanted to know how to support them best.

Putting my feelings into words and seeing how others were similarly affected began to heal my mind and give me the strength to get through.

I remember lying on the acupuncturist's table the following week, praying. The things I said to God took me by surprise. Usually, I would lay there and say, "Please, God, let this baby be our miracle," or "Please let us have a healthy baby soon," but that day, I found myself praying, "Thank you, God, for this experience. Thank you for everything we've been through and for the amazing opportunity for growth you've put in front of us."

If you had told me a year prior that I would be thanking God for all the heartbreak, loss, and challenges we'd gone through, I would have told you you were crazy. But there I was. Thankful.

# Chapter 8

# PSC Rears Its Ugly Head

## Spring 2017

In March 2017, I woke up to my phone ringing. It was the middle of the night, and my phone read, "Hubby." I rolled over and realized Reid wasn't in the bed next to me. I answered, confused.

Reid said, nearly in a whisper, "I'm sorry to wake you, but I need you. I'm really sick."

"Where are you?"

"On the couch," he replied through gritted teeth. I jumped out of bed and went into our living room to find him covered in multiple blankets and shivering uncontrollably. Reid was always hot, yet he had so many blankets on top of him that I wasn't even sure where they all came from. He looked up at me with pleading eyes and said, "I don't know what's wrong. My stomach hurts so bad I can't sit up, and I can't stop shaking. Nothing I do helps."

Reid had occasional flare-ups from the ulcerative colitis that would make him feel like this, but the symptoms were never this intense and usually didn't last this long. He had been in pain for three hours, hoping it would pass.

"Wait here," I told him. "We're going to the ER." I took the dog out, threw on a bra and some pants, and got us in the car. Reid doubled over in the passenger seat of my car, arms wrapped around his abdomen. The look on his face made me question whether I should call an ambulance instead of driving the seven minutes to the nearest ER. I turned on my hazard lights and ran every red light on the way to the hospital.

I pulled up to the double doors of the ER. Considering his state, Reid got out and walked inside as quickly as possible. He couldn't stand straight, so he had difficulty walking, but we wanted to get him checked in as soon as possible.

I parked the car and ran from the parking lot to get inside. Out of breath, I burst into the waiting room and found Reid sitting in front of the reception desk, waiting to be checked in. The triage nurse seemed to be in no hurry, and I glanced around at the mostly full waiting room – it was apparent others had been waiting quite a while, and some were even asleep.

I explained to the triage nurse that he was in intense pain and had been like this for three hours. I pleaded with her to help him and get him seen quickly, but we were told we'd have to wait.

We found seats in the waiting room, and I felt so helpless. Reid's face contorted as the waves of pain flooded his system.

By the time they took Reid back to an exam room, I was speaking on his behalf. His pain had become so excruciating that he couldn't even talk. This is a guy who sat on a burst appendix for ***three days*** before going to the hospital (before we were together, I must add,) so I knew his pain had to be beyond terrible.

Once back in the exam room, I explained that he had primary sclerosing cholangitis and ulcerative colitis, and his pain may be a result of one of those chronic illnesses. I urged them to call his gastrointestinal doctor, Dr. Reddy, to get his thoughts on what may be happening. I begged them to give him something for the pain. Anything. Just do something. Now.

As many of us know, though, the ER never moves as quickly as we hope – especially in the middle of the night. They couldn't give him pain medicine until they ran some tests and knew what they were dealing with.

As much as I tried to respect the team, their lack of urgency frustrated me. I paced the room and often walked to the nurse's station to inquire about what they would do next and whether they had called his doctor. My logical brain knew they were doing what they could, but I couldn't just sit there and watch my husband like that.

Several hours later, the ER team managed to get Reid's pain level down from a nine to a seven. They had also spoken with Dr. Reddy, who deduced he was having a cholangitis attack. He had a severe infection in his gastrointestinal tract, and it would need to be treated as quickly as possible, or it could be fatal. They started Reid on an intense round of antibiotics and tried a different painkiller to attempt to get the pain in a tolerable range.

They admitted him to the hospital and said Dr. Reddy would be in shortly to see him.

By the time they wheeled Reid up to his hospital room, he was borderline septic. The bacteria had entered his bloodstream, which made the situation even more volatile. The medical team told us an infectious disease doctor would also monitor him.

Dr. Reddy came to see him that morning. He offered a reserved smile when he entered the room and quickly got to business. He warned us that this meant Reid's disease was progressing, but he wasn't sure yet to what extent.

With an active infection, they did not want to perform any procedures. Doing so may have led to more complications and could have given more life to the bacteria already wreaking havoc on his system. They would check on his liver once things cleared, but treating the cholangitis was the priority. The doctor told us Reid would be in the hospital for several days to make sure the infection wasn't continuing to spread.

Shortly after Reid was admitted, I had an intrusive thought: *I should be ovulating later this week, so our chances of pregnancy this month just went out the window.* I had convinced myself I was not going to obsess over it… but it was always in the back of my mind. My husband lay in the hospital bed, and while I worried about him and his well-being, I was also concerned about missing out on our chance to be pregnant that month.

After a couple of days in the hospital, they were able to get Reid's pain under control, and it seemed the antibiotics were working to help kill the infection. Reid stayed in the hospital for five days, and I didn't know it at the time, but that event was priming us for what lay ahead.

Before they discharged Reid, they placed a PICC (peripherally inserted central catheter) line in his arm to administer more antibiotics through an IV at home. The PICC line would need to stay in for two more weeks, and they taught us how to change the bulb on the end of the line twice a day. We had a follow-up scheduled with the infectious disease doctor so he could keep an eye on the infection.

Dr. Reddy mentioned that once the cholangitis cleared, Reid would need another spyglass cholangioscopy (a direct examination of the bile ducts using a tiny scope.) We were familiar with the procedure since Reid had already been through several. I called Dr. Reddy's office to schedule the appointment, assuming the infection would be cleared when Reid had the procedure since it was several weeks away.

Reid and I volunteer at the Houston Livestock Show and Rodeo every year. It is a huge event, and our volunteer team has four dedicated shifts. Reid was an assistant captain on his volunteer team, so he needed to be onsite if possible. He left the hospital just in time for us to make the first shift. The PICC line and bulb of antibiotics didn't stop my husband from volunteering.

Reid had difficulty standing for the long periods the shift required, but he had great support around him. His teammates helped him get through the shifts without pushing his body too much. Most of them encouraged him to go home and rest. But Reid had committed to this and was determined not to let his team down.

We made it through the rodeo, and Reid got his PICC line out two weeks after he left the hospital. According to the infectious disease doctor, the infection seemed to have cleared, and he felt better. We were still unsure of what this meant as far as his disease progression, but we hoped that in a few more weeks, we'd have some more answers.

But before that time came, Reid landed back in the hospital. Either the cholangitis never fully cleared, or it had returned. Regardless, it was not good. He was in intense pain again, so back to the ER we went.

This time, we knew exactly what it was, so they were able to get him admitted and treat him quickly.

This was obviously not good news regarding his liver disease. The spyglass procedure would closely examine the disease progression, but that appointment was still a few weeks away.

Dr. Reddy came to Reid's hospital room the morning after he was hospitalized. He pointed out the obvious: these last two episodes indicated that the disease was progressing much quicker than we'd hoped. Despite the risk, the doctor decided he needed to go in and see what was going on, so they scheduled a spyglass procedure for the next day.

And here we are, back at that awful day I described in the prologue of this book.

After the spyglass procedure, Dr. Reddy said Reid needed to be added to the transplant list and that he had a 90+% chance of developing cancer without a transplant.

I couldn't believe the words I heard, and looking back, I feel I had an out-of-body experience that day.

When they diagnosed Reid, I assumed that *maybe* 10-15 years down the road, we *may* have some hard conversations. But here we were, only three years after his diagnosis, and Dr. Reddy was saying the things I hoped he never would.

Over the last three years, I think I had focused so much on our infertility and pregnancy losses that I avoided seeing how sick my husband was getting. I had been living in denial that his disease was substantial and that he would ever have to have a transplant. I downplayed it. I avoided thinking about it. His parents moved to Houston six months before this *because* it was evident to them Reid's disease had been progressing quicker than anticipated.

I later learned that Reid's mom saw a picture I posted of him on Facebook almost a year prior and gasped. He was so gaunt with dark circles under his eyes, and his skin was pale and yellow. That day, she and Ric started planning to put their house on the market and move closer to us as soon as possible.

Yet, I still refused to see how bad it was.

With the infertility and pregnancy losses, I could see it and feel it. I could research and join support groups. I blogged about it. The fertility doctor had laid out a plan for me. Sure, there was still a lot of uncertainty and waiting, but at least there was a plan.

There was no plan laid out for the progression of Reid's illnesses—especially the primary sclerosing cholangitis. We were told from the beginning there was no way to know how quickly or how much it would progress. When he was first diagnosed, Reid worried he would make me a widow. That had never been a thought of mine until that day in the hospital.

I had been pushing so hard to have a family with this man, who I loved so much, but I avoided the reality that he may not even be around for the family we had been fighting for. But now I couldn't *not* see that fact. Everyone around me thought it, but no one would ever say it. And when Reid did mention his concerns a few times, I brushed him off. I thought he was over-dramatizing the situation. In hindsight, I just couldn't let my brain go there. Living in denial was more manageable than realizing I might lose my husband and that there was nothing I could do about it.

Once Reid settled in his hospital room and he and I had a good cry together, I walked out to the front entrance of the hospital. I sat on the bench outside the hospital doors and started making calls. I may have lived in denial for the last three years, but I just had my wake-up call. This would not be the end of our story, and I was going to make sure of that.

I called several of our family and friends to share the latest news. I was in tears for the first few calls as I explained the doctor's findings. I had to catch my breath several times. The information we had just received was still sinking in, and it terrified me. Then, I felt like I shifted into action mode and started presenting the facts.

One conversation I remember distinctly was with Nate, one of Reid's best friends who lives in Indiana. He said, "What can Angie [his wife and also a good friend of Reid's] and I do to help?"

I replied, "Just come visit. All anyone can do right now is be there for him." Nate assured me they would, but he also asked if he could contact Indiana University Hospital in Indianapolis. He knew they had a transplant program, and he wanted to connect us with any resources he could. He wouldn't accept the "just be there for him" comment because that's not who he is. We are blessed to have several of those people in our lives. It helped to know he would also not accept defeat and would be there fighting alongside us.

The next day, I called the J.C. Walter Jr. Transplant Center at Houston Methodist Hospital to start the transplant evaluation scheduling process.

# Chapter 9

## Transplant Evaluation and Listing

### Spring–Fall 2017

For an entire week or so after that day in the hospital, I felt completely overwhelmed. I went to bed with my head spinning and woke up with it spinning. I didn't get much sleep. We faced a huge unknown and had so much to learn.

Reid and I were aware that organ donation saves lives, and we were both already registered donors, but we didn't know anyone first-hand who had received an organ transplant. Everyone around us had questions that we couldn't answer just yet. Neither of us felt comfortable or functioned well without having the answers.

Reid felt better once we got home from the second hospital stay. During his spyglass procedure, Dr. Reddy stretched his bile ducts, which would allow the infection to fully clear. We were on edge for the first few days because his fever spiked every couple of hours. He was exhausted, as his body was still working hard to clear the rest of the infection.

A week after Reid's hospital stay, we drove to the Texas Medical Center to meet with a hepatologist who specialized in liver transplants. When we walked into his office, he greeted us with a smile and got right down to business.

"Are you okay if I record this conversation on my phone?" I asked him.

"Sure."

"Thank you. We are very overwhelmed, and I want to make sure we hear everything accurately." I pushed the record button on my phone and held it between us and the doctor.

The doctor reiterated that there is no cure or treatment for PSC, and a liver transplant was his best (only) option at that point. He didn't think Reid would have a problem getting listed, but the challenge would be that he wouldn't be placed very high on the list.

For liver transplants, the patient is placed on the list based on their MELD (Model for End-Stage Liver Disease) score. The MELD score uses a combination of creatinine, bilirubin, INR (international normalized ratio for prothrombin time to predict three-month survival), and sodium to determine where you are on the list, and the score can range from 6 to 40.

Despite how bad Dr. Reddy said Reid's bile ducts were, his actual liver hadn't felt the full effects of the disease yet. His bile ducts were extremely scarred, which was causing him to have cholangitis attacks and increasing his chances of cancer, but his liver wasn't damaged as badly. You can't replace the bile ducts without replacing the whole liver. At least not with today's technology.

At that appointment, we inquired whether Reid would be able to get a transplant if he did develop cancer in the bile ducts – cholangiocarcinoma. The answer was a big *maybe*. It would depend on where the tumor was in the bile ducts, what stage, and the aggressiveness of the cancer. The *maybe* answer made us feel a little better since our assumption going into the appointment was that a cancer diagnosis would remove him from the transplant list. This doctor shared that there were more options than we realized if we did end up with a cancer diagnosis.

We were glad to have answers and start the process of getting on the list, but it would still be a big waiting game. Our wait for a family, along with the disappointment that frequently came with it, had, in a way, prepared us for the wait for an organ transplant.

We inquired about how long the wait was for a liver transplant, but the doctor couldn't answer. It depended on many factors, and Reid had extra challenges with his low MELD score (when he was very sick in the hospital, his MELD was still only a 16). We asked about being listed at other centers in addition to Houston, and he encouraged us to do so.

The transplant list is divided into regions, with many different areas across the US. Each region has its own "list" and average MELD score, which it uses to determine who gets transplanted. We figured Reid might have a better chance of receiving a transplant sooner if he listed in a different region since the Houston area's list was quite long and had a high average MELD score. Those that were being transplanted in Houston around that time had MELD scores closer to 35, which was incredibly high.

Reid was evaluated at J.C. Walter Jr. Transplant Center in the Texas Medical Center a month after his hospital stay. During the two-day process, we met with a financial counselor, a cardiologist, a dietician, a transplant surgeon, a hepatologist, a nurse practitioner, a transplant coordinator, and a social worker. All those people made up the transplant team. Reid had 20 vials of blood drawn, a bone density scan, an EKG, a panorex scan, a chest x-ray, an echocardiogram, a carotid Doppler, an MRI, and a pulmonary function study. It was a lot.

Not only did they have to make sure his body could withstand a transplant, but they also wanted to be sure he could mentally tackle the challenge ahead and would have a solid support system to help him through it. They were also requiring him to make some dietary and lifestyle changes to support a transplanted organ.

We welcomed the opportunity to learn as much as possible about the process, and we both felt as ready as we could be for what lay ahead. The intense process overwhelmed me and calmed my nerves all at once. It intimidated me, but we were doing something. We were moving *forward*.

During the listing process, we sat in the waiting room at the transplant center next to a bench covered with colorful tiles. I began reading the tiles as we sat there. The bench was made to honor those who died and became organ donors, and their loved ones decorated the tiles for them.

Tears rolled down my face, and goosebumps covered my entire body as I read each one – a father, a sister, a grandfather, a child, a mother. These incredible people saved lives and impacted countless others by becoming organ donors. We were there because we needed someone to save my husband; we needed a hero and a family to think of others in their time of sorrow, just like the ones on the tiles had.

I had been so focused on the actions needed to get us here that I hadn't allowed myself to think of what it meant to receive an organ transplant. One person dies, and their choice to be an organ donor can allow several others to live.

I remember sitting there, experiencing a mixture of feelings… sadness for those who lost their loved ones, but also hope that we all have the opportunity to impact others in such a massive way after our death. I prayed for the families of the organ donors, and I hoped their gift of life helped them through their grieving. I also prayed for an organ donor to save my husband one day soon.

The transplant team mentioned there may be a possibility that Reid would be listed as "low MELD in need" on the transplant list. This would mean that Reid could get a subprime liver - a "B" liver instead of an "A" - but it could work. The reason a liver is classified as a subprime can vary, but it doesn't mean it's bad. It just means they don't think that the liver will do well in a very sick and dying patient. Reid was 31, otherwise healthy, and had a great chance of recovery after a liver transplant. He should be just fine with a subprime liver. We were hopeful this option would help him get a liver quicker.

A few weeks later, they listed Reid on the transplant list in Houston with a MELD score of 11, which is extremely low. He was not able to be listed as "low MELD in need" just yet, but his transplant coordinator mentioned they would continue to try to get him classified as such.

In Houston, at that time, they were transplanting patients with MELD scores in the mid-30s, which meant the person was very sick and likely admitted to the hospital while waiting for the transplant. With so many things working against us, it seemed Reid would never have a high enough MELD score to get transplanted before he developed cancer.

Shortly after we learned about the extra challenges we would face in getting Reid a transplant, I had a conversation with my boss, Julie. She had been there for me all along, and as I explained the process, Julie said to me, "Abby, this is your job now." She could see the obstacles before us and knew I needed to dedicate all my time and resources to saving my husband.

I stepped back from my full-time position at the company and dove into my new role. I reached out to others in similar situations and spent most of my time researching and calling other transplant centers. I appreciated that we had the privilege to take on such a task when many others didn't have that option.

We felt we were in a race to get him transplanted before he developed cancer in the bile ducts. Cholangiocarcinoma has an incredibly low rate of survival, which terrified us.

Within a week of being listed in Houston, I contacted Indiana University Hospital in Indianapolis via the contact Nate had found for us. I learned they were transplanting people with a MELD score in the mid-20s. The odds were much better that Reid could receive a liver transplant sooner there than in Houston.

We scheduled a transplant list evaluation in Indianapolis for August, which was just a month away.

We attempted to make the most of the trip to Indiana by scheduling time with Reid's friends who still lived there. We felt some relief having another option available, but we also felt a little frantic and sad that we were at a point where we thought we needed to seek out all the options.

We spent some quality time with Nate and Angie, which was good for the soul but also had an underlying feeling of doom for me. We weren't there because we just wanted to hang out; we were there to evaluate my husband for a liver transplant. Only three years into our marriage, we were there to save his life.

While in Indianapolis, we sat in an educational class about transplantation with their center. A couple behind us kept bickering and complaining about how long the class took. We were all there to save the lives of our loved ones, and they were arguing. At one point, the husband complained loudly to his wife, and she said to him, "Well, you're the one who had to go and get sick!" I couldn't believe what they were saying, and I remember thinking it was unlikely he would even get listed for transplant with the attitude they both had.

Reid and I laughed about her comment, which became our running joke. Once in a while, I would say to Reid, "Well, you're the one that had to go and get sick!" when we were dealing with a challenge, making us both laugh. That joke reminded us we were *not* that couple… we were in this *together*.

Our meetings with the transplant team in Indianapolis gave us great hope. They thought Reid might be able to get exception points on the transplant list, which would place him higher and possibly get him a liver sooner. When we originally scheduled the meeting at Indiana University Hospital, we were under the impression that if he were listed, he would be considered inactive until we relocated to Indiana. To receive a liver, you must be within 3.5 hours of the transplant center.

But as we talked more with the transplant team, they decided to keep him "active" since there were many direct flights from Houston to Indianapolis every day, and if the donor were on life support, it would give us time to get to the hospital. We were all hopeful he would get the exception points when they listed him, so our outlook had changed significantly. Based on the conversations in the meetings, he could get a liver within a few months in Indiana, which was a massive shift for us.

A few weeks later, we learned Reid was added to the transplant list in Indianapolis, but he did ***not*** get the exception points as we had hoped. At that time, the criteria for exception points required him to have been hospitalized three times. He had been hospitalized twice. Frustration and defeat set in as he sat so low on both lists. My research continued, as did my desperation to figure out how to get my husband a liver quicker.

Our plans to build a family were constantly nagging in the back of my mind. Some people probably wondered why I even worried about that, considering the news we received for Reid. But because of that news, I think I was more worried.

We had to anticipate things no one ever wants to think about. Reid worried about leaving me a single mother. I felt that if he did leave this earth sooner rather than later, I would be comforted having a "piece" of him here with me. I wouldn't want that reality for anyone, but it was our reality. Despite everything we were going through, I couldn't imagine us not having a family, but this also meant our fertility window got smaller. With my AMH as low as it was and Reid's health spiraling downward, I didn't feel time was on our side.

We scheduled a meeting with our fertility doctor, where we laid everything out and discussed our options. We were trying to avoid IVF because of the significant cost (we needed to save every penny we had for Reid's health), but here we were. We decided to freeze Reid's semen. If he were to get cancer soon, there was a good chance he would be sterile after treatment.

It made me feel better knowing we had that backup and a plan going forward.

# Chapter 10

# IVF – Here We Go

## Fall 2017

After three years of trying to create a family and three pregnancy losses, it was time for In vitro fertilization (IVF). We started the process in August of 2017, the same month we traveled to Indiana for Reid's transplant evaluation.

Several factors played into our decision to finally start the IVF process:

- My low AMH would continue to diminish more with age.

- It had been over six months since we conceived the old-fashioned way.

- All three of our spontaneous pregnancies ended in heartbreak.

- IVF would allow us to test the embryos before we transferred them to my uterus. Given that two of our pregnancies had chromosomal issues (both completely different issues), it became vital for us to be able to do the PGS (Preimplantation Genetic Screening) testing to ensure the embryos were compatible with life.

- IVF would also give us more control over the timing – if that was such a thing, which we needed with the wait for Reid's liver transplant. We also weren't sure what the anti-rejection medications would do to Reid's fertility once he received a transplant.

During this time, I continued pushing forward but did not fully process everything happening.

My mom started a fundraising campaign to help us cover the costs of both IVF and Reid's liver transplant. We also began selling shirts with *Expect Miracles* on the front and *A Grateful Heart is a Magnet for Miracles* on the back. The shirts symbolized hope and allowed others to rally around us during this time.

Over the next few months, we raised over $10,000 to help offset the cost of IVF.

We sold almost 700 shirts and often got pictures of others – even strangers – wearing the shirts to encourage us along our journey. *Expect Miracles* can be applied to so many different situations. The two messages on our shirts spoke to me during our wait, so I had hoped they would also help others, but I never imagined it growing into a movement the way it did. It warmed my heart to know we were going into this with a tribe, and each time I received a picture of someone wearing one of our shirts, it filled me with so much joy.

At first, I had a heavy heart that we had reached this point. When we made the tough decision to start IVF the year prior, we had come to terms with it and then found out we were pregnant on our own the day before we were to begin the process. In my mind, I hoped and prayed it would happen again. But it didn't.

Reid had been on board with IVF far longer than me. He saw IVF as less of a risk since it would allow us to check the chromosomes of the embryos through PGS testing. To me, it meant admitting defeat. And quite honestly, the process scared me to death. I don't like shots (I mean, who does?), and I didn't like the idea of pumping my body full of hormones. The concept of spending $20,000+ to maybe get pregnant felt terrifying. I also didn't like the odds of only a 60-65% chance that it would work; if it didn't, we'd have to start all over again.

But there we were. Surprisingly, I felt at peace once we started the process. We had a teaching appointment at our fertility clinic, where they showed us how to inject the hormones and explained everything. It didn't completely overwhelm me like I thought it would. I left the clinic thinking, "Okay, I can do this!"

Our IVF "stimming" process was as follows (stimming is the act of stimulating the ovaries by adding extra hormones to produce more eggs):

- I was prescribed oral birth control for two weeks (it ended up being a little longer for me because we had a hurricane hit Houston, and our clinic was closed).

- I completed baseline bloodwork and an ultrasound to ensure my hormone levels were where they needed to be and to confirm that my ovaries and uterus looked okay.

- Once given the all-clear, injections started a few days later.

- We did 10-12 days of injections between 6-9 PM. For our first round of IVF, we had one injection each day that consisted of two medications we would mix. These medications, Menopur and Gonal-f, increased the size and number of the follicles in my ovaries, which would produce an increased number of eggs.

- During this time, I had bloodwork and ultrasounds every two or three days.

- As the follicles grew, my body would try to ovulate to release the eggs. Cetrotide, another injectable medication, was added to keep my body from ovulating. This additional medication was used for five to six days.

- Once we had good-sized follicles (around 18 mm), they set up my egg retrieval appointment. After that appointment was set, they gave me a specific time to take my trigger shot.

- The trigger shot was scheduled for exactly 36 hours before the egg retrieval. This shot causes the body to ovulate 36 hours later.

- The egg retrieval is an outpatient procedure where they put me under anesthesia to extract the eggs from my ovaries.

- They then fertilized my eggs with Reid's sperm (which he brings in a cup – the guys get off so easy… ha, see what I did there?!)

- The day after egg retrieval, we would know how many eggs were fertilized and became embryos.

- Five to seven days later, we would know how many embryos made it to freeze.

- They would then take samples of each of the embryos to send off for PGS testing.

- Once we got the test results back, a week or two later, we would know how many (if any) healthy embryos we had.

I felt nervous about the shots and bloodwork, and Reid worried about the fact that I would be pumped full of hormones. Considering everything we were dealing with, I couldn't blame him.

When we went to pay for the IVF medication, we were surprised to find our insurance company covered that part of it. We added that to the win column.

The first week of IVF was tough. But not for the reasons I expected; I felt so tired that I could fall asleep while standing and drinking a Frappuccino. And Reid was right to be worried about the hormone rage… it proved to be intense.

Throughout our first round of IVF, we were thrown some curveballs, which seemed pretty standard for us.

We started the injections on Sunday, September 3rd, and they weren't as bad as I'd made them out to be in my mind. The needle we used to inject the medication into my abdomen was only a half inch and 27 gauge (which is tiny). The medication burned as it went in, but I learned that my right side didn't hurt nearly as bad as my left side. Fortunately, they wanted me to alternate sides each night, so it only hurt every other night—another so-called win.

I started the process on 225 IUs of Menopur and 225 IUs of Gonal-f. I prepared all the medication each night, iced my stomach, and then Reid would inject. I liked having him be a part of the routine (plus, I didn't have to look at the needle as it went in). I'm not sure he was so happy to be the one stabbing me each night, but he did it.

Four days after starting the injections, I went in for my first transvaginal ultrasound and bloodwork. I walked away super discouraged. During the ultrasound, they couldn't find my ovaries. Yeah, you read that right. They couldn't find them.

I have a retroverted uterus (my uterus tips backward), which we learned during my previous pregnancies. But what I learned during this ultrasound was my tilted uterus also makes my ovaries harder to find; they tend to hide.

We couldn't measure the follicles in the ovaries since we couldn't find them on the ultrasound. The nurse assured me this was not a huge deal because my ovaries would enlarge when the meds started working, making them easier to see.

Later that day, the nurse messaged me to tell me the doctor had reviewed my bloodwork and I needed to increase my dosage to the maximum amount. *Great, so my body wasn't cooperating all the way around.* That night, I increased my dosages to 300 IU of Menopur and 300 IU of Gonal-f.

When we went to pick up the extra medication from the specialty pharmacy, we were surprised to learn our insurance company only covered the medication the first time, not if you needed to order more mid-cycle. So, we paid $2,500 for a few days of medication. The blows kept coming.

Two days later, I went in for another ultrasound and bloodwork. Reid went with me this time since I was a mess after the last one.

When the nurse walked in, I said, "I hope you're prepared to work today because I'm not leaving this room until you see my ovaries." She did work a little harder than the nurse on Wednesday, and she found them. But then came the next blow.

We had two follicles in the right ovary that were 8 mm and one that *may* grow in the left ovary. That's quite a low number of follicles. Follicles are the structures in which eggs grow… each follicle will hopefully produce one egg. This result meant we were looking at maybe two or three eggs they could potentially retrieve. I should have been happy we had any, but I couldn't help but be disappointed. Since my AMH was very low, they didn't expect a normal number of eggs to be retrieved, but I had been hoping for more than just a few.

I spent the rest of the day mad at the world, and sad things never seemed to go right for us. Everyone on the road that day was called a bad name, like the worst names.

I went to my acupuncturist appointment, and when he shut the door, I burst into tears. I had sat in that room days after two pregnancy losses and told him that I'd lost babies, but I had never cried like this. Fortunately, he specialized in infertility and had grown to know me quite well over the past year, so he said all the right things. He assured me it only takes one; we only needed one healthy embryo to make a baby.

I noticed he added needles in places he normally didn't: on my ears and across my forehead.

I said, "You don't usually do those."

He replied, "Yeah, I know…" with a little smirk.

He was trying to "acupuncture" the crazy out of me.

I heard from the doctor's office later that afternoon, and they wanted me to start the Cetrotide injections the next day. That at least meant we were on the right track timing-wise. This medication keeps you from ovulating while your follicles continue to grow. I added that to our nightly routine on Saturday night... one shot of Menopur/Gonal-f mixture and one shot of Cetrotide.

Adding the Cetrotide made me nervous. I heard from others that it might burn a little more, and now this meant I would be doing two shots each night. My heart started to race as it got closer to the time to do the injections. I had gotten into a routine with the other medication, but now we were stepping into another unknown. Sure, it was just one more shot. But it was **one more shot**. *What if it hurt so bad that I couldn't continue?* My skin crawled just thinking about it.

When I went to mix the Menopur and Gonal-f, I had a full-on freak-out. I swear the Gonal-f pen dumped in twice the medication than it was supposed to, even though the odds were unlikely it would malfunction like that. I called my nurse (she probably regrets giving me her cell number), and she convinced me it was okay and that I should take the dosage.

After I got off the phone with her, I questioned it all over again. I yelled at Reid, "JUST TELL ME WHAT TO DO!" He suggested I take the already mixed dosage and used math to support his argument. I chose to squirt it down the drain—a full dosage—probably $700 worth of medication literally down the drain.

After that, we got ready to take the Cetrotide, and Reid saw a giant air bubble in the syringe. He started to say he needed to get the air bubble out, but I started yelling again. "DON'T TELL ME ABOUT THE AIR BUBBLE. YOU'RE MAKING ME MORE NERVOUS!! JUST FIX IT!!" I screamed and cried.

What a fun Saturday night.

As the process continued and I took even more hormones, the crazy continued to get worse. One day, something minor triggered me and made me angry. I told my best friend, "I could just cry right now. And I don't even know exactly what I would be crying about, but I feel like I am about to cry."

A few days later, I talked to my mom, and she urged me to look at the positives when I just needed to vent. I got so mad at her that, in my hormonal rage, I decided to "punish" her.

The following day, I had another ultrasound and bloodwork appointment. They saw three potential follicles, which we hoped would produce at least two healthy embryos.

After that appointment, my mom texted me to see how it went. I waited a full hour to respond to her. Take that, Mom.

# Chapter 11

## First Egg Retrieval

### Fall 2017

On September 16th, 2017, we had our egg retrieval. I believed things would work out for us, but I also tried hard to manage my expectations. I knew only a few eggs would be retrieved, but I hoped they would be healthy, moving us one step closer to our baby.

Reid and I got up extra early that morning. I wore my *Expect Miracles* shirt and a pair of fun socks I had ordered for the day that said *Retrieve. Believe. Conceive.* Before we left the house, Reid made his "contribution" into a cup, which we then placed in a white paper bag. I held the bag tightly for the ride to the surgery center as if it were liquid gold.

My nerves were on edge, and my thoughts raced with excitement. Something was happening. We made it to a retrieval day, which I thought might not happen when they couldn't find my ovaries on that first ultrasound.

As we walked into the waiting room of the surgery center, my body tensed. The last two times we were here, we were having a D&C to remove a pregnancy that was no longer thriving. As much as my brain tried to set those emotions aside, my body remembered.

I nervously handed the receptionist the bag with the cup. She knew what was in the bag, but I felt the need to tell her so she would be sure to handle it as carefully as I had. She assured me she would pass it off to a nurse and handed me paperwork to complete.

The last few times I had sat in that waiting room resulted in gut-wrenching pain and heartbreak, so I scanned the room for a seat that wouldn't bring on more déjà vu than I could handle. "Let's sit over here," I told Reid as he followed me to the corner opposite where we had been on our previous visits.

I looked around at the couples in the room and wondered whether they were there with hope or sadness—likely a mix of both.

After I turned in the paperwork, a nurse called me back and instructed me to remove all my clothes and put on a gown. "I will be right back in to start your IV, then we can bring your husband back," she said.

Once Reid was brought back, the nurse talked us through the process. Then, the doctor came by to check on us before they took me back for the procedure. The doctors at our clinic rotated for the egg retrievals, so I didn't have Dr. Griffith, but I had heard good things about this doctor.

As I walked into the procedure room, my entire body began to tremble. My stomach tightened, and my breaths came quicker. *This time is different,* I reminded myself. *You are not here for the same reason as before.*

I climbed onto the table and was asleep shortly after.

As I woke up in the recovery room, the doctor came to my bedside and told us they had retrieved four eggs. Reid and I were elated, and I high-fived the doctor. We had more than one. The eggs were in the lab being inseminated with Reid's sperm, and we would get an update on them within 24 hours.

The next day, we learned that two of the four eggs had been fertilized. We were still in the game. The two embryos just needed to continue to grow and survive several more days before they could perform a biopsy and freeze them.

Those days of waiting seemed to go by so very slowly. I had stepped back into working part-time since we had Reid listed at a couple of transplant centers, and we were in a holding pattern. Working on some big projects kept my mind busy during that wait.

Almost a week after my egg retrieval, we got a call that our two embryos had made it to day six and would be biopsied and frozen. We were ecstatic that both of them made it, even if it was a day later than the typical timeline for IVF. The embryologist took a sample from each of the embryos to be sent off for PGS (peimplantation genetic screening) testing, and then they were placed in a freezer as we awaited the results. They said it would be one or two weeks before we received a report.

While we waited for the results of the PGS testing, Reid had another spyglass procedure to check on the status of his PSC. We were seeing a different doctor than the one who diagnosed him, but we had developed a great relationship throughout many appointments with him. Dr. Raijman was familiar with primary sclerosing cholangitis and was head of Gastroenterology at the hospital where he worked. Dr. Raijman and Dr. Reddy worked together to ensure they didn't miss anything, which gave us extra comfort.

We drove to the medical center early that morning for the spyglass procedure and stopped at Starbucks on the way there. Reid couldn't eat or drink, but I get *hangry,* and nobody wants that.

I brought a notepad to work on a blog post while I sat in the waiting area. Blogging had become therapeutic, and I knew it would help me process my thoughts as I waited. We had already gone through several of these procedures. They had become pretty standard, and we had our routine down. I even knew what Reid wanted for lunch after the procedure and planned to pick it up on the way home.

Once they finished, Dr. Raijman called me back to the procedure room. Reid was still sedated, lying on the bed in the middle of the room. Dr. Raijman's team started prepping him for recovery and then wheeled him out on a gurney.

The doctor had a serious look on his face. He shared his concern about possible malignancies. Reid's bile ducts were incredibly scarred, and time was of the essence. "We need to exhaust all possibilities to get him a liver sooner," he said. Dr. Raijman explained that he would make sure he reflected in his notes the severity of Reid's disease progression so that we could hopefully apply for exception points on the transplant list. It seemed exception points were the only thing that would bump him up the list to get him a liver sooner.

There had been a slow but steady progression of the PSC since Reid had been put on the transplant list. Others noticed his physical changes, and our friends and family were worried. Living with Reid and seeing him daily, I didn't notice the difference in his appearance until I saw us in pictures. His eyes had become sunken in, and he had lost a lot of weight. He felt tired all the time, and his skin itched like crazy. But he did his best to push through it all and went to work each day like normal.

After Dr. Raijman announced his latest findings, we felt stuck. Our doctors said Reid needed a liver as quickly as possible. However, according to the guidelines set forth by UNOS—the United Network of Organ Sharing—Reid wasn't sick enough to get a liver anytime soon. We were fighting an uphill battle. We hoped the notes from Dr. Raijman would allow for exception points, but after being denied twice before, we weren't super optimistic.

The next day, I had a meeting at a client's office. I had become very close with this client, Steve, and he knew everything we were going through. He was like a work dad for me: always asking how things were going for us and offering to help in any way. Because of his support, I knew I could still meet with him despite the weight of the day before. Steve would understand if my head was a little out of sorts.

As I pulled into the parking garage at his office, my fertility clinic called. I answered to hear my doctor's voice on the other end, "Hi Abby... this is Jason Griffith. Did I catch you at an okay time?" *Shit. This can't be good,* I thought. *Please don't let this be bad news about our embryos. Please, Lord, let everything be okay.*

He told me he was between surgeries but had just received information he wanted to share with me immediately. "I really hate to tell you this, but both of your embryos came back abnormal." My entire body tensed, and the floodgates opened.

I had previously heard that embryos can come back as abnormal but still have a chance to correct themselves after transferring to the uterus. I asked him if that was at all possible with these. He didn't think so, but he didn't have the specific chromosome details in front of him. I begged, "I desperately need hope. Please give me some hope." But he wouldn't give false hope, and I sensed from his voice that this round was over without anything to show for it. I could tell he sincerely empathized with us.

Dr. Griffith told me he would send my nurse a message so she could follow up with more specifics about the embryos, but he was so sorry to be delivering bad news to us once again. We hung up, and then I sobbed in my car so loudly that I'm sure everyone in the parking garage heard me. *Why did everything have to be so damn difficult?*

I called my client, told him the news, and apologized, but I couldn't walk into the building in that state of mind. He understood and said he would be thinking of us.

On the way home, I called Reid. Every imaginable emotion I held escaped all at once. I was furious, broken-hearted, disappointed, anxious, and absolutely tired of feeling that way.

Reid called the clinic to see if he could get more information about the embryo issues. Even though Dr. Griffith made it clear they would not be able to be used for a transfer, we still wanted more information. I think both of us were holding out hope there was some mistake or that there was some way one of those embryos was compatible with life.

Our nurse returned his call quickly and shared that one of our embryos was a male with an extra 4th chromosome—Trisomy 4. Our other embryo was a female and was missing one of the 13th chromosomes—Monosomy 13. They would not transfer either embryo as they did not believe they would be successful. Our first round of IVF was officially over.

We had so many questions:

Do we do another round of IVF?

Could we even afford it?

Do we only make *abnormal* babies? Is there a way to fix that?

Do we need to look into embryo adoption or egg donation?

Will we ever be parents?

And if we do become parents, will Reid even be here to see his kids grow up?

We scheduled a meeting with Dr. Griffith, hoping to get some answers to our questions. We walked into the fertility clinic feeling so defeated. Reid and I were convinced he would not suggest doing another round. Considering our low numbers and testing results, we thought it was a lost cause.

But to our surprise, our doctor held onto the hope we had lost. He felt that some tweaks to the medications could produce better results. He laid out his plan of what he thought would work better, encouraging us. Unfortunately, IVF can be trial and error. Everyone's body works differently and responds to different medications, so it's hard to know what will work best until you try it.

I loved that our doctor didn't just give us a standard, "Here's what we do next." Instead, he carefully considered what my body might need and personalized his plan for us.

We went straight from his office to the financial counselor's office to figure out what it would take to get through another round. Once we met with her, we learned that we could afford another round of IVF, especially with the support others had provided to us during the fundraising campaign my mom had set up. The fertility clinic also gave us some discounts since we never made it to transfer with our first round.

We agreed to try for another round and prayed this time would work better than the last.

# Chapter 12

## It's... Just... Too... Much

### Fall 2017

A few weeks later, we heard from Dr. Raijman's office. The biopsies they had taken during Reid's last spyglass procedure had come back benign. We were grateful they couldn't find any cancer, but also still worried it may be there hiding or would develop soon. We needed the doctor's notes on the findings to apply for exception points on the transplant list. They were our golden ticket and the key to getting Reid a transplant before it was too late.

I felt as though I was walking around with a pit in my stomach. My anxiety soared, and I couldn't figure out how we would end up making it through all of this.

We were getting ready to start round two of IVF, and while it contributed to my anxiety, IVF was more of a "known" challenge.

We had been through it once before, and we knew what to expect regarding the process.

Now, I was concerned because of the unknown of what would happen to my husband. There were times when the possibility of him not being here would creep into my thoughts, causing my entire body to ache and nearly taking me to my knees. Without him, it felt like nothing else really mattered.

I'm not saying that infertility and pregnancy losses were the lesser of our struggles. There is no comparison. Each struggle had its significant challenges, affecting me differently depending on the day.

Four weeks after Reid's spyglass procedure, after calling the nurse again to ask if they were ready, we finally received the notes from Dr. Raijman. The nurse asked if I wanted her to read them to me before they sent them to our transplant centers, and I said yes. I sat listening intently as tears welled up in my eyes. The notes were *very* direct.

The doctor had told me in person about the possible malignancies, but I think I was still questioning whether I heard him right.

Dr. Raijman's notes read: "I have discussed with patient and wife, at length, as well as with other involved physicians, that he has cholangioscopic features highly suggestive of malignancy. While at present, it has not been pathologically demonstrated that he has cancer, he is at a very high risk for developing cancer. The last digital cholangioscopy revealed more advanced mucosal changes in areas not identified during previous cholangioscopies, thus further supporting the evolution of his disease likely to cholangiocarcinoma. His only therapeutic option is liver transplant, which should be done as soon as possible."

To hear the nurse read the notes directly from the doctor about possible malignancies and just how much his disease had progressed shocked me to my core. I became inundated with mixed emotions, both sorrow and hopeful desperation. The matter-of-fact statement that the transplant centers would be receiving confirmed our reality, yet it also carried the hope of a brighter future ahead.

I had to come to terms with the fact that my husband might develop cancer in his bile ducts before he received a liver transplant.

* * *

It was October, and we went to a Halloween party with some friends a few days later. My emotions were still raw. I stood there looking at my husband and became painfully aware that I could lose him. My face flushed, and tears filled my eyes as I watched him talk and laugh with our friends, pretending things were *normal.*

While the other couples in the room were ordering new furniture for their home or discussing how to decorate their nursery, we were dealing with the likelihood of cancer and praying my husband would get a new liver before that happened. I wondered whether we could ever discuss a nursery as confidently as they were.

One of our friends mentioned how his wife hated that she couldn't have a drink since she was pregnant. Rage flooded my system as I barked back at him, "Reid can't drink either. For completely different reasons."

I ran to the bathroom just as the uncontrollable sobs escaped. Their guest bathroom was right off of the main area where everyone was gathered, and I prayed that no one could hear my sobs as I cupped my hands over my mouth to muffle the sound. No one truly understood what we were going through, but could I blame them? The heartache consumed me.

We also recently learned that Reid's sister was pregnant with twins, which was a wonderful blessing, but if I'm being completely honest, it filled me with jealousy.

Some days, it all just made me so angry. *Why were we dealt such a crappy hand?* Infertility and the pregnancy losses weren't enough;

now, we were fighting for my husband's health, which included a new liver for him. And I mean **fighting**.

I had been on the phone with different doctors and transplant teams more times than I could count. The transplant coordinator in Indianapolis knew me by my first name... I could call and say, "Hi, it's Abby," she knew exactly who I was and all about my husband's case. No other couples we knew of were dealing with the same struggles. We were that couple for whom everyone felt sorry. And I hated it so much.

Saying the right thing to someone going through difficult times can be challenging. People don't realize how their words can affect a person's well-being, and I experienced this firsthand and often. I felt I needed to educate those around me to better understand how hurtful some of their comments were. I didn't want others to feel like I did. The alternative would have been to avoid people after they made those comments, but their friendships were more important to me than that. Those uncomfortable moments drained me.

Reid had been putting on a brave face in front of others, but he could see the emotional distress it put on me. I think he worried more about how it was affecting me *mentally* than how it was affecting him *physically*.

Dr. Raijman's findings were sent to our transplant teams in Houston and Indianapolis, so we were stuck waiting to hear back. The transplant team at IUH applied for exception points for Reid, but Houston did not. In Houston, exception points still wouldn't have gotten him in the range of getting a liver sooner. We were blessed to live in a city with one of the best medical centers in the world, but because so many patients traveled to Houston from all over the country, they had a longer waitlist than most other areas in the US.

If Reid were awarded the exception points in Indiana, we would likely relocate there with the hope that an offer for a liver would come soon. If he didn't get the points, we would move forward with our second round of IVF.

Ready for the shocker? We heard back that, yet again, they denied him the exception points.

We began to realize he may never be awarded exception points to move up the transplant list. It felt like we were in a race where the finish line kept getting pushed further and further away, and we kept getting injured as the race continued. But we weren't giving up.

I regularly contacted the other transplant centers and doctors, determined we would find a way.

# Chapter 13

# Second Egg Retrieval

## Winter 2017

While we waited for a liver, we shifted our focus back to IVF. In November of 2017, we started round two. This time, they began by putting me on testosterone for 21 days. Dr. Griffith was trying a completely different protocol, which gave us hope that we'd get different results.

While I was up for anything and wanted to trust what the doctor thought would be best for us, I do not recommend adding extra testosterone to your system when you're already stressed. It had me raging, and it was a little scary. The most minor things would set me off, and everything became a much bigger deal than it usually would be. I was driving on the highway one day, and another car started to come into my lane. I swerved to avoid them but then over-corrected and almost hit another car. My hormone-overloaded nervous system made it feel like I had no control over my body. In addition to the rage, this protocol called for five daily injections. It was a lot, but we were determined to make it through this process again.

Despite the medications' side effects, round two seemed to be going much better than round one.

We made it through the stimming process without significant challenges, and they retrieved *seven* eggs. That was huge for us and a much higher number than we expected. All seven were fertilized.

This was it; we were finally progressing on our journey to start a family. However, as the days went on, some of the embryos slowly stopped growing, and on day six, we got a call letting us know we only had two embryos. It was disappointing, but we had two. It wasn't zero. *Please, Lord, let at least one of these embryos be healthy.*

The embryos were biopsied and frozen. The samples were sent off for PGS testing, and we prayed hard that this would not be a repeat of the last round.

A couple of weeks later, we got a call from Dr. Griffith… once again, the embryos were ***both abnormal***. Rage and bitterness flooded my entire nervous system. I couldn't believe it. He couldn't either.

Why did it feel like everything was constantly stacked against us? These embryos had different chromosome abnormalities than all the others. They were Trisomy 16 (an extra 16th chromosome) and Monosomy 22 (missing one of chromosome 22). It didn't make sense.

We met with Dr. Griffith shortly after we received the results; he was as confused as we were. Why would six different chromosome issues show up? Two of our pregnancy losses had chromosome issues, and all four of our embryos had them as well, but they were all different. It may have given us some answers if the same chromosome was affected, but that wasn't the case.

During our meeting with him, we asked about egg quality, sperm quality, and additional testing. Whatever we could throw at him, we did… we were grasping at straws. Unfortunately, they couldn't do much more testing than we had already done. The only thing that *may* give answers was to have Reid see a urologist and do a few more tests. Those would help give us a better look at the genetic constitution of Reid's sperm, but they also have huge margins of error and were a bit unreliable. But trying to get more answers was worthwhile. Dr. Griffith referred us to a urologist, and we agreed to reevaluate after the test results.

I continued doing my best to hold onto any ounce of hope I could. That weekend, I had an arrow tattooed inside my left wrist to remind me to keep pushing forward regardless of the setbacks. I found a quote about an arrow that resonated with me: "An arrow can only be shot by pulling it backward, so when life is dragging you back with difficulties, it means it will launch you into something great. So focus and keep aiming."

There were days when I felt our story would not end happily. And then there were days when I just knew in my soul that the ending would be more incredible than I could even imagine—that's the feeling I had to hold onto.

One afternoon, while running errands, I got a text from a friend. It was a link to a song he had heard and felt he needed to send me. The song was *Miracles* by Unspoken. I clicked the link while sitting in my car in a crowded parking lot. I sobbed as the song blasted through the speaker of my phone. The song held the overall message to keep praying for miracles regardless of the setbacks, and the words left me with chills all over my body.

In moments like that, I felt so surrounded with love and support that I thought we could survive anything.

I needed to trust that this wasn't where we'd be forever and that better things would come our way. I feel like our support system and my faith helped me to have that perspective in the middle of all the adversity. Don't get me wrong, I was a mess most days. I often would pull over in parking lots to sob as my best friend sat on the other end of the line, listening to my cries and pleas for things to get easier. But I knew I couldn't stay there. I had to fight for our future and my husband because both were absolutely worth fighting for.

One of my friends from our fertility support group shared the book *It Starts with the Egg,* which discussed ways to improve egg quality and overall quality of life by eliminating toxins and changing your diet. I read that book cover to cover and went on a mission to rid our systems of as many toxins as possible. I'm sure Reid thought I was crazy. In fact, I know he felt that. But he also knew it was my way of trying to have some control over the situation.

I replaced our pots, pans, food storage, and products in our shower. All of our candles got thrown out, I swapped out most of my beauty products and did my best to eliminate processed foods. Reid and I agreed we would try this for three or four months, and then we'd try for one more round of IVF. Getting rid of toxins and eating better would hopefully also help Reid's health, so we had nothing to lose with this plan.

We would focus on what we could and see what the next few months had in store. As we rang in the New Year for 2018, I held onto so much hope that this **would** be our year.

# Chapter 14

## Directed Organ Donation

### Winter – Spring 2018

One night in February, just before 1 AM, I received a Facebook messenger call from a friend in my hometown. Reid and I both woke up, but I assumed it was an accidental dial, silenced it, and fell back asleep.

Suddenly, I sat straight up in bed, feeling like maybe it had been an intentional call. I checked my messenger app to discover several messages from Jennifer, the person who had called, saying she knew of a family who was keeping their grandson on life support so that he could be an organ donor. She wondered whether Reid could potentially use his liver. My heart nearly leapt out of my chest, and I was instantly wide awake. I immediately called her and gave her the information she needed to pass along.

The family was going to attempt a directed donation to Reid. We knew very little about directed organ donations. Jennifer told us the family spoke with their doctor, who told them as long as the potential recipient was on the list, no matter their place, they could receive a directed donation if the organ was a match.

Jennifer was very familiar with our story; my family had known her for years, and she was very involved in the community in which I grew up. She followed our updates via my blog and Facebook page, and her family prayed for us through our journey. Jennifer immediately thought of Reid when she heard the family was looking for organ recipients through friends and family.

Chills covered my body as I thought about how incredible it was that she saw the opportunity and reached out to help us. But, that poor family. My heart broke for them thinking about the tough decisions they had to make. What an absolutely amazing thing they were doing.

It felt like a dream. Reid and I lay in bed, wide awake, unsure what to do. Should I pack a full hospital bag? No, we didn't know for sure. Should we start alerting our family? No, too early for that. Should we call our transplant center and warn them? I tried, only to get the answering service.

How does this even work? What can we do to ensure this offer comes through? I posted in a Facebook support group for PSC to see if anyone else had gone through this before, but I didn't get much help there since it was the middle of the night.

I decided to let the system work as it should and wait for the hospital to alert our transplant coordinator.

Still in bed, we talked about the potential. We knew this wasn't a guarantee Reid would get the liver, but we were sure he'd at least get a call to come in and start the testing process to see if he was a match. We cautiously held onto optimism, which was unusual for us at that point. We turned our phone ringers up and tried to get a couple more hours of sleep.

Morning came, but no phone calls. I called our transplant coordinator around 10 AM, and she informed me they hadn't heard anything either. We remained confident but realistic, not knowing how this particular situation usually worked. Reid and I were hopeful we'd get a call any minute.

Unfortunately, we received a text from Jennifer at 11:30 AM stating a miscommunication at the hospital, and the liver was matched with another recipient. The family expressed their apologies through Jennifer that Reid wasn't the recipient.

This family had just removed their loved one from life support and donated his organs to save the lives of others, yet they were apologizing.

Reid and I were more disappointed than we thought we would be. We never imagined an opportunity like this, but it didn't set us any further back than we were the day before. Reid was still alive, and we were able to keep fighting for a liver for him as they mourned the loss of their grandson, son, and friend. My heart hurt for them.

This opportunity opened our eyes to another potential way for Reid to receive a liver, which encouraged us for the future.

Around this time, I also got a call from the dad of Reid's best man at our wedding. He is a dentist in St. Louis and knew our story well. Their whole family had been following along and supporting us through the process. He had dinner with a friend who is an OB-GYN and shared our story. It turns out this doctor's daughter had the same disease as Reid, and she had a transplant a few years earlier. They had gone through a lot of the same challenges we had in terms of moving up the transplant list, and he wanted to help us in any way he could.

The next day, I spoke with his friend, Dr. Super, and he and I talked about several of the larger transplant centers across the US. He vowed to help us figure out how to get Reid a liver sooner and offered to also be a sounding board if we needed any advice on the IVF front. This kind of support surrounded us during those difficult times, and I will forever be grateful for all the incredible people we were connected with during our journey.

After reviewing the list of transplant centers with Dr. Super, we agreed it would be best to get Reid evaluated at Emory Healthcare in Atlanta, Georgia. They seemed to have a lower average MELD score for liver transplants, so we thought he could get a liver there quicker. I contacted them and discussed the process with their transplant intake coordinator.

Emory scheduled Reid to be evaluated for their transplant list in July of that year.

# Chapter 15

# More IVF Planning

## Spring 2018

We began getting more insight into our fertility journey in the early months of 2018, which sometimes only led to more questions. We met with a urologist in January, and he ran three tests on Reid: a semen analysis, a DNA fragmentation test, and a sperm fish. Then we waited - and waited and waited - for the results to come in. Of course, they weren't conclusive once we finally got the results, which meant we had no black-and-white answers. Our urologist then referred us to a genetic counselor.

The genetic counselor reviewed our history along with the results of the testing we did on Reid, and she concluded that we *may* both have issues contributing to the chromosome abnormalities. But there's no medical proof of that.

Reid's semen analysis and DNA fragmentation test came back normal. The sperm fish, which checks for abnormal chromosomes, returned *slightly* abnormal. Of the 500 sperm they tested in each category, one to three were abnormal. This didn't directly indicate a problem but showed there *may* be an issue.

The genetic counselor said we could certainly try IVF again but advised we shouldn't expect different results than the last two rounds. I felt deflated after that appointment.

Reid and I scheduled an appointment with Dr. Griffith for the following week. We had decided we would likely go for another round of IVF to "check the box" (at least, that was my feeling). I wasn't optimistic another round would work, so I figured we'd be headed toward the next step in our journey of creating a family (either embryo adoption or infant adoption). We both wrestled with our feelings about the future.

After we consulted with Dr. Griffith, Reid and I walked out of there surprised and scared. We sat in his office, and I started rambling about all that had happened over the last few months and what the other medical professionals had told us. The look on his face wasn't one of discouragement or defeat, as I expected it to be.

I quit rambling and asked, "So, what's your opinion? What do we need to do?"

He looked at both of us and said, "I think we need to go forward with another round of IVF and **not** test the embryos."

*WHAT?!?! Is he kidding? We've gone through so much testing, and all of our embryos have had abnormalities. Now, he wants us to forgo testing?!*

I tried to remain calm on the outside as my internal dialogue was screaming. I looked at Reid and could see his mind was blown. We smiled at each other, and I sensed an unspoken "we're still in the game" confirmation between us. I sat there reeling from the conversation as my stomach fluttered and hope flooded my body.

Let's talk about PGS testing for a minute. It's definitely imperfect.

You can get "abnormal" results that may produce healthy babies. The test takes a sampling of the embryo to test the cells, so it may grab some abnormal cells, but that may not reflect the embryo as a whole. It is also possible for an embryo to correct itself over time and be completely normal. It's widely debated in the fertility community.

Reid and I originally fit the "criteria" of a couple who should use PGS testing, considering our two chromosomally abnormal losses. This is why we tested with both previous rounds of IVF, and the results showed a different abnormality each time. Our doctor thought those *could*, in fact, potentially be normal embryos. But because we had the testing done and they'd been deemed "abnormal," we were afraid to use them for a transfer.

We sat there a little stunned but also very pleasantly surprised. I fully expected to come out of that appointment having the same conversation we had with the genetic counselor. The three of us discussed Dr. Griffith's plan, and we (mostly Reid) asked many technical questions. It felt like we were taking a giant leap of faith moving forward, but we both felt we needed to take it.

We completely trusted our doctor. He had been there with us for all the ups and downs of pregnancy losses and infertility. He knew our full story (even the latest on Reid's health) and always considered our entire situation when making suggestions. He explained the risks, and it would be a huge unknown. He said he understood if we weren't comfortable with taking that step.

*But this could be precisely what we need to start our family.*

In the second week of May 2018, we started the process for round three of IVF.

The doctor changed our protocol once again based on new research. This protocol consisted of higher dosages of Menopur and eliminating Gonal-f, which he recently learned had been more successful for patients with low AMH, so we felt good about the changes.

I started the testosterone priming once again, preparing for how it would make me feel, but knowing that this time, I was at least aware of how the medication affected me.

# Chapter 16

## The Fear or Hope of Cholangiocarcinoma

### Spring 2018

The following week, Reid had another spyglass procedure. I had lost track of how many he'd had by this point. We knew from the last one that his chances of developing cancer were high. However, his blood work hadn't changed drastically, and he hadn't had any cholangitis attacks in the previous year, so we were hoping that meant we weren't there yet.

Reid's mom and my mom offered to attend the appointment with us, but neither Reid nor I thought it was necessary. We assumed it would be a similar update to the last one, where the doctor reminded us that Reid needed to get a liver as quickly as possible.

I sat in the crowded waiting room, Frappuccino on the small end table next to me, expecting a day for good news. I looked around at the other families and could feel the sense of worry in the room around me. I wasn't worried, though; we knew what to expect. We had been here, and I felt confident I knew what the doctor would say today.

Once the procedure was done, a nurse called my name. I quickly grabbed my purse and drink and followed her back to a procedure room where Dr. Raijman was sitting by a countertop with his laptop open. I looked for his usual bright smile that could light up the room, but he did not have a smile on his face. He briefly greeted me, then showed me the pictures he had taken inside Reid's bile ducts. He looked me in the eye and said, "If I showed these pictures to one hundred other doctors, every one of them would say Reid has cholangiocarcinoma. *All one hundred.*"

This was the exact reason we were racing to get him a liver transplant. But at that moment, my heart sank into my stomach, and it felt like we lost the race. My face flushed, and my hands felt clammy as I stood there listening. My drink suddenly felt heavy, almost slipping through my sweaty palms. Dr. Raijman said he would send off the biopsies and we'd know more in a few weeks, but we needed to exhaust every possible option to get Reid a liver transplant as soon as possible.

Cholangiocarcinoma (bile duct cancer) is very aggressive, very hard to detect, and has a very low rate of survival. It is so hard to detect that Dr. Raijman said even if the biopsies came back benign, the likelihood of cancer remained. We hoped this would be the winning ticket to bump Reid up the transplant list with exception points so he could have a transplant soon. How crazy is it that we actually *hoped* the biopsies came back malignant?

The team wheeled Reid to recovery, and my unstable legs led me back out to the waiting room alone, regretting not taking either of our moms up on their offer to join us for what was supposed to be a routine procedure.

I found one of the only seats left in the waiting room and took a few deep breaths to calm my nerves. I called Tinker, Reid's mom, and asked her to grab his dad so I could share the update with them together. I could hear her carry her phone to the next room to get him. *Why do I have to be delivering bad news again?* I felt like I broke their hearts a little more each time I provided an update, and I could do nothing to make it all better. I took a few more deep breaths and rubbed my sweaty palms on my jeans. *You can do this, Abby. You've done it before, and you can do it again.*

Once Reid's parents were both on the phone, I relayed the update while using every bit of strength to hold back my tears, pausing a few times to catch my breath. I wanted to be sure I didn't forget anything the doctor had told me. Tinker's voice cracked as she asked questions to ensure she fully understood. I knew she felt just as helpless as I did. I imagined the ache she felt in her heart, knowing her son's health continued to decline.

After that heartbreaking exchange, I called a few other family members and close friends to share the update. Then, the nurse came to take me back to the recovery room. She pulled back the curtain as Reid pried his eyes open and gave me a half smile. I tried once again to crack a few jokes to keep it light. Surprisingly, it became easier this time… I had been by his bedside with life-altering news before, and I knew I could hold it together until he was ready to hear the update.

When he finally came out of the anesthesia enough for me to share the information, I scooted my guest chair closer to his bedside. I whispered the latest update to him, feeling like I was making it all up. Surely, I had heard Dr. Raijman wrong.

We sat silently on the 40-minute drive home, reeling from the information we had received and unsure what to do next. A dense cloud of distress consumed the air around us. The doctor's words kept replaying in my head as I tried to figure out how I could have misheard Dr. Raijman. Reid called his parents from the car. We knew they would want to hear his voice even if the anesthesia hadn't fully worn off.

Silence loomed in our house that afternoon. We sat staring at the TV, broken, feeling the blows that kept coming and shattering our hopes and dreams.

I decided to do a video update that evening to share the information with those following our story. Typing out the words felt impossible, but getting the news out there seemed necessary in hopes that someone might offer a glimmer of hope. I sat on our bed and recorded the entire update, feeling like I was having an out-of-body experience while sharing the doctor's findings. I presented the information matter-of-factly and managed to hold it together the entire time. After sharing the update, I lay on the bed for a while, searching my incoming messages for a sliver of hope and encouragement.

With the latest news, we decided to try to move up the listing appointment at Emory Hospital in Atlanta. I called their transplant team to relay the update. Their intake coordinator said if we could get a note from our doctor saying the appointment needed to be expedited, they could work us in sooner. We originally planned to go there in July, but that was two months away, and we both knew we didn't have time to waste.

I emailed Dr. Raijman that night, and by the next morning, I had been copied on an email from him to the transplant hepatologist at Emory stating Reid needed to be seen as soon as possible.

That next day, Emory rescheduled Reid's listing evaluation for the last week of May, two weeks away. This new date posed a problem because I would be starting injections for our third round of IVF that week and couldn't travel because I needed to be monitored by my fertility doctor.

To be listed for an organ transplant, you have to show the medical team that you have a strong support system to help you through the process, and you must bring your support with you to the listing appointments. I had been at every appointment before this, and the thought of not flying to Atlanta for this wrecked me. But we had already started the process for this round of IVF, and if we scrapped it now, we would not only be out the money we paid but would also have to wait another month or two before we could start again.

Time to pivot and call in the backups.

Reid's best friend, Nate, who lives in Indianapolis, had been requesting another way to help, so we asked if he could fly to Atlanta to meet Reid for the appointment. Without hesitation, he said, "Yes."

Reid met Nate and his wife Angie the following week in Atlanta for the listing appointment. Denise came to stay with me to help with appointments and injections. I didn't *need* someone there with me, but it helped ease the weight of all we had going on. Plus, it meant I got to spend some quality time with my best friend and her kids, who I also claimed as my kids.

I received regular updates from Reid on his testing at Emory. Having been through the listing process at two other transplant centers, we were quite familiar with all that it entailed.

Meanwhile, I started the IVF injections for round three. The process was going well despite Reid's absence.

I had been blogging often to share updates on our current situation, and the blog was reaching far more people than I ever expected. A nurse practitioner contacted me from a transplant center in Alabama because she heard our story and wanted to help. She connected us with the transplant surgeon on her team, and he began reviewing Reid's case.

As Reid wrapped up his testing at Emory, they said they likely wouldn't list him there. By their standards, he wasn't sick enough to be listed for a transplant. We knew his MELD score remained low, as he had extra challenges with PSC that put him low on the transplant list, but we were incredibly disappointed that they wouldn't even list him. The Emory team planned to review his case further after we sent additional information from Reid's doctors, but it didn't look promising.

In addition to all this new information, we learned Reid's biopsies had come back benign. We didn't celebrate that news because it meant he would not be moving up the list to receive his transplant sooner.

There we were, standing in quicksand up to our armpits; everyone around us wanted to help, but no one had a rope to save us.

# Chapter 17

## Third Egg Retrieval, First Embryo Transfer

### Summer 2018

After Reid got home from Atlanta, I had another week of injections and then my third egg retrieval. Since we weren't testing the embryos, we had agreed with our doctor to try for a fresh transfer.

A fresh transfer meant that five days after the egg retrieval, we would transfer an embryo(s) into my uterus. We had yet to complete the transfer process, so this was a significant next step. Reid and I were hopeful we would finally get pregnant and give birth to a healthy baby.

During this egg retrieval, the doctor retrieved six eggs, five of which were fertilized. The team watched the embryos grow, and then they scheduled me for an embryo transfer on day five.

On June 14th, 2018, we again arrived at our fertility clinic's surgery center. The drive to the clinic had gone from one filled with dread to one filled with hope and eagerness.

We were unsure if they would transfer one or two embryos, and we had no idea how many (if any) had even made it overnight. I had a full bladder for the procedure, as instructed by the doctor. So full that I had to pee a few times before the procedure even started. I took the assignment seriously.

Dr. Griffith walked into the prep room and shared that we had two embryos at the morula stage. My stomach fluttered with faith and optimism. Ideally, they wanted to see the embryos at the next stage - blastocyst - before they were transferred. Blastocyst embryos are more mature and have marginally better chances of success than morula embryos. Since we had two morulas and zero blastocysts, he suggested we go ahead and transfer both.

My heart skipped a beat as I thought about the potential outcome.

I always wanted twins, but after everything we had been through, I needed to be mindful of wishful thinking. I smiled at Reid, and he responded with a nervous smile. I sensed his thoughts: *Twins? Are you sure we're prepared for that?*

We agreed to transfer both embryos.

Dr. Griffith said he would see us in the procedure room shortly and left to visit the next patient. The nurse pulled the curtain back to the prep area, handing Reid a sterile "Marshmallow Suit" to wear over his clothes, a bouffant scrub cap, and booties to cover his shoes. She then gave us paperwork to transfer two embryos and said she would be back soon. We signed the documents, Reid suited up, and the nurse escorted us to the procedure room.

As we walked in, they had me climb onto the table. I placed my feet in the surgical stirrups, and they tilted the table up and back. There was a screen to my right, and Reid stood on my left, near my head. Dr.

Griffith walked in and joyfully greeted everyone. He joked with the embryologist and nurse, then looked at Reid and me and said, "Let's get you guys pregnant!"

The embryologist brought over a catheter and showed Dr. Griffith the accompanying paperwork. He stated the two embryos belonging to Timothy (Reid) and Abby Gray were ready for transfer. After confirming the necessary information, we all watched the screen as the catheter went through my cervix and into my uterus. He pushed a button to release the embryos and then pulled the tube back out. The tiny specks stayed in my uterus where he had placed them.

My body calmed as if it had just been filled with joy, and then I shivered. We finally got to an embryo transfer, and I had embryos in my uterus. The next step – we wait. I closed my eyes and said a little prayer that they would stay right where they were as they wheeled me back to the recovery area.

The calmness and bliss stayed with me that day. Reid felt he needed to be a nervous wreck to counterbalance. My confidence with this transfer had me feeling we'd celebrate a pregnancy soon.

Dr. Griffith strongly advised bedrest for three days post-transfer, so we were prepared to camp out on the couch for the next few days.

Reid analyzed every little symptom and became very alert to how I felt. Whenever I got up to use the restroom, Reid asked where I was going or what I needed. Finally, I said, "I'm going to pee… is that something you can help with? If you could figure out how to make that happen, I would love that."

The day after our embryo transfer, we received a call from our clinic. I assumed they were checking on me, but surprisingly, she said, "I'm calling to update you on your embryos." *Update on our embryos???*

We assumed the two we had transferred the day before were the only two surviving embryos. The situation hadn't sounded promising that the others would grow to the point where we could freeze them, but she told me we had TWO additional embryos make it to freeze. Amazing! We thought this would be a one-and-done transfer. Now, we had two beautiful embryos waiting for us.

After hanging up with her, an intense sense of happiness washed over me. We had more chances and received some good news, which amplified my optimism.

I had bloodwork and a clinic visit four days after the transfer to check my progesterone and estrogen levels. The clinic had me taking both of these hormones to increase our chances. My levels came back within normal range; whew. In every pregnancy up to that point, we always had to add more hormones.

A few days later, however, the story changed. My hormone levels dropped, so the doctor increased my progesterone dosage. They were still within "normal" range, but both numbers had dropped 50%.

The PTSD set in immediately, and all positivity vanished. With each of our three pregnancies, this is where things went downhill. My hormone levels would drop, and we would supplement with more hormones, but eventually, it led to the inevitable. That is not always the case with everyone – I had heard plenty of stories where women just needed to be on extra hormones, and they were fine. For us, however, our history had proven otherwise.

My anxiety kicked into overdrive as my heart raced, and I tried to catch my breath. The internal spiral began. *This wasn't going to work. Would we ever have kids? Would I be able to survive another heartbreak?* I tried to remain positive, but I felt doing so was pointless after all we had experienced.

Reid and I were supposed to leave for vacation with my extended family the next day, but I decided I couldn't go and experience more pain. My cousin and his wife were pregnant, and I didn't think I could bear to sit and look at her pregnant belly all weekend. After my big pity party, Reid and I agreed we would rethink it all in the morning. "I think we should go, but not if it will be a detriment to your mental health. I will absolutely follow your lead on this," he told me.

Thursday morning, I woke up believing things would work out. This had to be our miracle. I needed to stay hopeful and push through. So much of our support system had good feelings about this transfer— it would work. We packed our bags and agreed we would not miss another event due to the never-ending roller coaster we seemed to be on.

We enjoyed our family vacation, but there were also moments when my thoughts would take over, and I would retreat to our vacation home bedroom. My family floated the river on Saturday, and Reid and I stayed back at the house. I wanted to take every little bit of caution not to jeopardize the success of my transfer.

When we arrived home on Sunday, I took a pregnancy test. Negative. That brought me down, but I still had a grip on our dream. I had read on Dr. Google that some women who got negative results ten days after transfer (which was where we were) went on to have healthy babies. Certainly, that would be us. It just had to be.

As I opened my eyes Monday morning, I was overcome with anger as I thought about the most likely outcome of this situation. Later that day, I had an appointment to check my hormone levels, and I felt I knew how things were going to play out. We would be getting bad news yet again.

That entire day, I sulked around the house, carrying the heavy pit in my gut. Reid came home from work around 10 AM to be with me. He was worried about me and wanted to be there when the call came in.

I went into the bathroom to dig the pregnancy test out of the trash and take a picture (because, you know, that's what {crazy} people do), and there it was – a faint line. I couldn't believe it. *Did I miss that yesterday? Or did it get darker after I threw it in the trash?* Suddenly, a spark of hope appeared. The faint line probably meant it wasn't great news, but I began to pray... hard.

A couple of hours later, my nurse called and said, "We did go ahead and test you (for pregnancy). Your levels are low, but they're there. Let's see you again tomorrow, and we'll be able to tell you more then." So, we were pregnant... but again, we had to wait and see if the seemingly unavoidable would happen. I grasped onto hope with the tightest grip. For the rest of the day, I kept praying and pleading, *God, please let this be a healthy baby. Please let my numbers go up. Please let this be a healthy baby.*

I underwent more bloodwork on Tuesday, twelve days after the transfer. Then, I attempted to keep myself busy until the call came in. My mind would jump from *We're going to get good news; this is just a slow start* to *Don't be stupid; you know this won't end well.*

As I walked into my acupuncturist's office around 2 PM, the nurse called and told me my numbers had gone down. She said the doctor wanted me to stop taking all medications and he would call me later that afternoon. There it was - another loss. This time, a chemical pregnancy, a very early miscarriage.

Pregnancy loss – 4, Healthy babies – 0

Reid and I were heartbroken, angry, and tired. So tired. Tired of being told "not yet," tired of sharing bad news, and tired of trying to look on the bright side all the damn time. I told myself it was okay to be sad and resentful. We had a right after dealing with all the heartbreak. But then we would pick ourselves up and keep going.

# Chapter 18

## The Continued Fight

### Summer 2018

A few weeks after Reid traveled to Atlanta, we received a letter from Emory Hospital. Reid's MELD score was too low, and they wouldn't even list him for transplant at their hospital. I knew that would likely be the answer, but as I read the letter, my frustration mounted, and I felt a surge of rage. This was becoming quite ridiculous.

Nate and I set up a website later that month to find Reid a liver. I designed shirts that read, "My {friend/husband/son/family member} needs a liver transplant," and prepared to place a car decal across my back window. Since we had learned about directed donation, we felt that was our best hope. A directed donation meant that Reid would get a liver "willed" to him by someone who was losing a loved one. Directed donation is a complex situation, but we were grasping at straws. We hoped the gift of life would provide hope for another family to see their loved one live on through Reid.

While Reid knew directed donation was likely our best bet, he wasn't ready for me to have the shirts and car decals printed. One day, as I gave him an update on what I had been working on, he said, "But that just doesn't feel right."

"What do you mean it doesn't feel right?" I snapped back.

"Why do I deserve to skip someone else on the list? How would it be fair for me to get a liver before anyone else?"

His questioning frustrated me, and I said, "Reid, I am fighting my ass off for you to live. I hope others have someone doing the same for them, but you cannot tell me to back down. I won't."

After that conversation, we agreed I would hold off printing any items. But if the next few weeks didn't have forward momentum, I planned to do whatever it took to get him a liver.

Another avenue for us to explore was a living donation. Dr. Raijman had always told us that a living donation was Reid's last resort. However, after his most recent spyglass procedure, benign biopsies, and no exception points, the time had come.

With a living donation, someone could donate a portion of their liver to Reid. The donated portion would grow to the size he needed, and the donor's liver would regenerate.

Our doctors originally believed this to be Reid's last resort for a few reasons. We did not have a living donor program in Houston then, which would mean traveling to another transplant center and sending friends there to get tested. Also, since PSC has a 40-60% chance of reoccurring in a new liver and is considered an incurable disease, the majority of centers in the US believed that it wasn't worth putting the donor through the risk of donating.

Fortunately, the data since then has shown that recurrence chances of PSC after LDLT (living donor liver transplant) are not higher than those who receive a transplant from a deceased donor. LDLT is now widely accepted for PSC patients, and Houston now has a living donor program.

The website we created for Reid provided information about how to directly donate a liver to Reid if anyone were presented with the terrible situation of losing a loved one. It also mentioned we would be working to get him listed with a living donor program, and anyone interested in getting tested should let us know.

As I've mentioned, I often shared our story on Facebook and Instagram. My Instagram was primarily dedicated to our fertility struggles, as there is an amazing group of infertility warriors on Instagram. I had also started talking about Reid's health there as well.

Once we completed Reid's website, I shared it on social media and had others share it as well. Then, I received an Instagram message from a nurse practitioner at Cleveland Clinic. She followed our story because she was also going through fertility treatments. She messaged me and explained she worked with the transplant team at Cleveland Clinic, which she shared has a fantastic living donor program.

Reading her message made me grateful that our paths had crossed, even if only through social media. I immediately knew this would be our next step. I called their intake coordinator and got the ball rolling to set up appointments in Cleveland.

That week, I received a phone call from Dr. Tate, a liver transplant surgeon in Alabama. Remember the nurse in Alabama who came across our story and shared it with her hospital's transplant surgeon? Dr. Tate was that doctor. He called me to discuss Reid's case and see how he could help. He had many questions, and at the end of the conversation, he said, "How can I best help you? Do you want me to be a resource and answer questions as you go? Do you want to come here to get Reid listed for transplant? What can I do?"

Moments like these helped to restore our faith and fueled my desire to continue fighting. There are so many good people in this world, and some wonderful people were reaching out to help us. I had been worried about putting our story out there, but by doing so, we were shown kindness and given more hope than I could have imagined.

In July of 2018, we packed our bags and headed to Cleveland. They had us scheduled to be there for almost a week for Reid's testing to be listed as a candidate for a living donation. Then, we would fly to Alabama to meet Dr. Tate and his team.

Reid had been having a lot of abdominal pains, so my anxiety kicked in, and I worried he would have a cholangitis attack while we were traveling. Any time we traveled, I researched the nearby hospitals, fearing he would need emergency medical attention. Of course, with this trip, we were traveling *to* hospitals, so we knew we were in good hands, but it still terrified me. What if he had a cholangitis attack while we were on the plane, and we couldn't get him to a hospital fast enough?

We tried to make the best of both trips despite all the underlying issues we were facing. We explored the area on days Reid wasn't completely exhausted from all the testing in an attempt to make it a vacation when we weren't at the hospital.

On our first night in Cleveland, we met up with Tiffany, the nurse practitioner who had reached out to tell me about their program. She kindly walked us through the process of living donation. We had immediately connected over Instagram when she reached out, and I felt that connection during dinner with her that night. We were so grateful to have someone so knowledgeable about the process. She made us feel as if we had been friends for years.

Meeting with the transplant team in Cleveland and having Reid do their required testing provided us with a light at the end of the tunnel. We had such a positive experience throughout the entire process with their team. Sure, we were a long way from Houston and our massive support system, but we weren't far from his hometown of Indianapolis. Plus, Reid had a cousin who lived in Cleveland with her family. Reid's parents planned to relocate to Cleveland temporarily if we took that route.

The surgeon at Cleveland Clinic told us Reid would be the ideal candidate for a living donor, and he agreed we were at that point. We still had concerns since living donation had always been our last resort. But at least we had that option. The word "cancer" had been thrown into the mix too many times, and we were determined to beat that clock.

The Cleveland team explained that an investigation into the potential cholangiocarcinoma was necessary before Reid could be listed. They requested an ERCP (an endoscopic procedure) with brushings and a FISH analysis (Fluorescence in situ hybridization — a laboratory technique that helps detect gene changes and chromosomal abnormalities that can cause disease). Wanting to minimize our time away from home, the team felt confident in our Houston doctor performing the procedure since we had an established relationship with him.

Cleveland Clinic wouldn't approve him for listing in their program until we got the test results, which would take a couple of weeks. If those results showed bile duct cancer, they would still likely list him, but it would change the process. Our overall plans would have to change, too, but we'd cross that bridge if we got there. Once approved, it would take two or three weeks for him to be officially added to their list, and then we could start testing potential living donors.

Cleveland Clinic had high success rates for transplants, and the way the doctors had talked about the process of living donation, along with Reid being an ideal candidate, made us feel confident.

When we had time away from the hospital, we enjoyed an Indians (now Guardians) baseball game with Tiffany and her husband and met up with Reid's cousin and her family. It felt good being there, and we were coming to terms with the fact that we'd likely be relocating to get Reid's transplant.

We left Cleveland and flew straight to Alabama to meet Dr. Tate. He and his team had been highly recommended, and they were ready to help however they could. Dr. Tate expressed to us that cancer or no cancer – our sense of urgency in getting Reid a new liver should be the same. He explained that Reid had multiple "dominant strictures" (narrowing in the bile ducts of the liver that prevent the normal flow of bile), and therefore, he needed a liver quickly. For that to happen, he felt we needed to get exception points. Here we go again. But Dr. Tate wanted to give it another try.

The one big problem was our insurance didn't cover the transplant center he worked with. Therefore, we had to start by appealing to our insurance and hoping they would make an exception and allow Reid to get listed there.

After all the travel, our next steps were clear: 1. An ERCP for Reid to get listed in Cleveland. Then, we could start sending potential donors to be tested. 2. Start working on the appeal to our insurance company to be listed in Alabama.

I posted our update on my blog and social media, and friends and acquaintances began reaching out to be tested. Most people who reached out weren't even in our close circle. This was an incredibly uncomfortable step for us, asking others to undergo surgery to save my husband.

Desmond, my friend from high school, contacted me through Facebook and wanted to be tested. He saw my post late one night and had spent the night researching. Reid and Desmond were the same blood type, so he just felt like this was something he needed to do. The two of them didn't know each other, so I suggested we have dinner so they could meet and he could ask any questions he had for us. We enjoyed our dinner with Desmond, and as we finished our meal, he said, "I'm in. Just tell me what I need to do next." Desmond's offer to get tested gave us faith.

Two nights later, we went to dinner with a couple we were friends with through the rodeo team we volunteered for. They had invited us out, and we always enjoyed hanging out with them, so we gladly accepted. At dinner, our friend Ray offered to be tested as well. Wow.

We had seen our support system come through in so many ways, and now we had others offering to undergo surgery and give Reid a portion of their liver. I don't think words can describe how this made us both feel.

# Chapter 19

## Embryo Transfer Round 2

### Fall 2018

On August 1st, 2018, we went in for a frozen embryo transfer. This time, we didn't tell anyone except our immediate family and very few close friends. We wanted so badly to be able to surprise everyone with good news. I also wanted to protect our hearts, and I didn't want to take the focus off Reid's transplant journey.

We had weeks of prep leading up to the transfer, which included oral estrogen and a nightly injection of progesterone in oil (PIO).

After the transfer, I truly believed it worked, and we were pregnant. All my hormone levels had been right in range, and my progesterone level came back higher than ever. *This had to be it.*

Our official beta hCG test (bloodwork to confirm pregnancy) wasn't set until Wednesday, the 15th. But, I was so confident it would be positive that I asked – well, begged – my fertility clinic to go ahead and test when I went on Monday. Reid and I agreed we would not be testing at home this time. We'd wait for the official test and let the clinic tell us. We knew that testing at home without having bloodwork to support it made me obsess over the darkness of the line.

One of my nurses called Monday afternoon and said, "Abby, I'm so sorry." *Really?? Are you serious?? But I had almost every pregnancy symptom in the book, and I was just so sure.* I honestly thought she had read the test wrong, but nope. The embryo we transferred had not implanted into my uterus, and we were not pregnant.

Reid and I were crushed again and feeling all the usual emotions. This was one of those days when I had a tough time seeing how we were going to get to the other side of this and hold a baby in our arms. The more "no" and "not yet" responses we heard, the harder it became to see the light at the end of the dark and winding tunnel.

I wished so badly I could say, "We're okay; I know this will work out." We had been through this type of disappointment enough times, so shouldn't we be used to it by now? Instead, bitterness and rage consumed me in the days after that news. I felt like a failure, and I let everyone else down.

I had put my body through hell to try to conceive a baby. I had prayed, begged, and cried more tears than I wanted to admit over the last four years of trying to start a family. We had endured countless tests and had injected hormones into my body over 100 times. I lost track of how many blood draws and transvaginal ultrasounds I had withstood. My husband and I suffered through four pregnancy losses, three egg retrievals, and two embryo transfers. Seriously, what more could we do? We were almost at the end of our rope, and I felt like our support system felt the same.

But we still had one frozen embryo left, so we were not totally out of the game. We prayed and pleaded that this last embryo would be our healthy baby. If not, we'd figure out where to go from there.

With a heavy heart, I reluctantly shared the news of our secret transfer, which ended in another disappointment. I didn't even want to post it because I felt guilty sharing bad news again. Still, I decided to share this message with our support system to tell them the best way they could support us, and I think it's important to share it here in case you know someone else going through something similar:

*We appreciate and need all the love, prayers, and positivity you have to spare. I know this saga seems to be never-ending. I am so tired of sharing bad news, and I'm sure you're tired of reading/hearing it. But as worn down as we feel and as hopeless as we may be some days, we still feel like we have to keep fighting for our baby. So, please check on us. Send us words of encouragement. Ask us to hang out. If you don't know what to say, it's okay to say so. Just let us know that you're there and behind us. You have no idea how much that helps. Please don't offer advice or make suggestions. I know we may seem crazy, but we aren't doing all this without great thought. And if this doesn't work, and we have to make more decisions, those will be just as tough. From the outside looking in, it may seem obvious what we should do next. But let me tell you, it's so much more complicated than that. And the decisions we make are not made lightly.*

At that point, I hoped that being an open book about our journey would help someone else not feel so alone. Sharing our struggles also helped me not feel so alone.

# Chapter 20

## Mosaic Embryos

### Fall 2018

Shortly after we learned our second transfer had not worked, we received a storage bill for the four frozen embryos from our first two egg retrievals. When I opened the letter, I looked at Reid, confused, "Our embryos are still on ice?"

"Our abnormal embryos? No, I'm pretty sure they were discarded," he responded.

"I'm holding a bill for another year of storage. They're still frozen."

We both looked at each other, unsure of what to say. We assumed these embryos had been discarded after learning they were all abnormal, but now we had to make a decision: pay $500 for another year of storage for the embryos or sign paperwork to discard them.

We had recently learned about mosaic embryos and were curious whether any of ours fell into that category. Mosaic embryos are usually deemed abnormal through PGS or PGT testing, but they are considered mosaic if the tested cells show both abnormal and normal cells. However, the test automatically defaults to an "abnormal" test result.

We found research suggesting mosaic embryos may have a chance to correct themselves or be normal and produce healthy babies. But there was also a chance they were indeed abnormal and would result in a miscarriage or significant birth defects.

Our fertility clinic didn't automatically tell us whether the embryos were mosaic, just normal or abnormal. We contacted the clinic to ask if we could discuss this in greater detail, and they referred us to a genetic counselor who could examine the abnormalities reported with each embryo.

A week later, Reid and I had a call with the genetic counselor. We sat next to each other on our couch, with the phone on speakerphone in between us. We asked many specific questions about the embryos and the abnormalities found. Some chromosome abnormalities were more likely to end in early miscarriages. Some were likely to have live births that would not survive.

The genetic counselor confirmed that with the abnormalities ours showed, she would not recommend transferring any of them. The big unknown was whether any of our embryos were truly mosaic because there might be a *slim* chance of them working. She had not received the mosaicism information with the PGS reports because we didn't know we had to ask our clinic to include it specifically.

Before we got off the phone with the genetic counselor, we all agreed on the parameters the embryos would have to meet to be transferred. Based on the data we discussed, the monosomy 13 was the only embryo we would consider transferring if it came back mosaic. Once she received the mosaicism information, we would all reevaluate.

After the call, Reid remained optimistic that one of those embryos could be mosaic and that we could transfer it alongside our last untested embryo. Reid secretly felt that an early miscarriage was something we had done and could handle again.

For me, the call confirmed the very, very slim chance any of them would work.

You could see the hope in his eyes as we hung up. He looked at me and said, "I really hope one of our embryos is mosaic."

My pulse quickened, and I developed a knot in my stomach. I countered, "Reid, I can't go through another miscarriage."

"I feel more comfortable with a mosaic embryo at this point. Especially if it falls into the category that we discussed of being okay to transfer," he argued.

I rebutted back, "I don't."

Memories of our past miscarriages came flooding in. This was his decision, too, but he didn't have to go through the physical part of a miscarriage, and I certainly did not want to go through that again. I felt transferring an embryo that had been deemed abnormal would guarantee a miscarriage.

"Let's talk about it when we get the results. It may not even be worth discussing right now." I shut down the conversation and we agreed to discuss it more once we got the mosaicism information.

# Chapter 21

# Embryo Transfer Round 3

## Fall 2018

I began taking oral estrogen and a nightly PIO shot in preparation for our final embryo transfer. Reid and I had agreed this would be our last round of IVF.

I felt confident we would only be transferring our last untested embryo since the conversation with the genetic counselor had pretty much solidified my thoughts that we wouldn't be transferring any of the abnormal embryos from the first two rounds.

We hadn't heard back since requesting the mosaicism information, and I had forgotten about it.

---

Desmond, our first potential living liver donor, was ready to go to Cleveland to be tested, so I had been working on flights and hotels for him. I focused on my to-do list and wasn't feeling the emotions of what we had in front of us. Some days, it's what I had to do to keep pushing through.

⸻

The day before our transfer, Reid called me on his way home from work and asked, "Did we ever hear anything about the abnormal embryos? Were any of them mosaic?" I told him I didn't think so. He kept holding onto this idea that one of those may be an embryo we would transfer, and I wasn't sure why, but it was important to him.

"Let me call the genetic counselor and see if I can catch her before she leaves for the day. Then I'll call you back," I told him.

The genetic counselor answered after a few rings. She had just gotten our results earlier that day and pulled them up to look. She said, "Well, you have one mosaic embryo. This one is monosomy 13, and it's a girl." My face flushed, and my body tingled with excitement.

One of the main reasons we agreed to transfer the monosomy 13 if it were mosaic is that if it was successful, we could do an NIPT (non-invasive prenatal test) at ten weeks pregnant. The NIPT checks for chromosomal abnormalities in specific chromosomes, and the 13th chromosome was one of those. Based on the research we did on the embryos we had, this embryo had the lowest risks if we were to transfer it.

I thanked her for the information and quickly got off the phone to call Reid back. As soon as he answered, I said, "The monosomy 13 is mosaic."

"We are transferring it, right? I feel like we have to." As much as I had been against transferring any abnormal embryos, he was right. I knew we had to take this chance, so we both agreed that transferring the mosaic was a risk we were willing to take.

I called our clinic to let them know we'd also transfer an additional embryo the next morning.

When I explained our plan to our nurse, she said, "I need you to come up here, like now, to sign paperwork. We need your signature before the close of business today in order to transfer this embryo tomorrow." I assured her I would be there within ten minutes, so she started working on the paperwork and said she'd have it ready when I got there.

On the way, I called a friend I had been really close with in high school. Amanda and I had grown apart over the years, but we had recently reconnected. She had been going through secondary infertility: she had one child but struggled to conceive her second.

Amanda and her husband had recently started the IVF process. She understood the ins and outs of IVF and the risks associated with transferring a mosaic embryo. I explained about the embryo and that we were planning to transfer it. "Are we crazy?" I asked her.

"Abby, I have chills. You know you have to transfer this embryo, and it's absolutely not crazy to take that chance. This could be your baby."

She was right, and the extra reassurance from her was just what I needed.

I walked into the clinic, and the receptionist greeted me with a smile. She knew Reid and me very well by then, and I felt like she and the entire team at the clinic were cheering us on every step of the way. She handed me the paperwork, which stated we were transferring an embryo deemed abnormal. Because of the extra risk associated with abnormal embryos (miscarriage, major birth defects), the clinic did not recommend transferring them. I signed the paperwork, saying it was our decision. I didn't even talk to my doctor about it; our minds were made up, and I don't think he could have changed them at that point.

The next morning - September 6th, 2018 - we woke early and headed to the surgery center for our final embryo transfer. This time, we did things a little differently. I asked Reid if my mom could attend this transfer, and he agreed. The three of us went to grab a quick breakfast on our way in.

We can be a little superstitious; by "we," I mostly mean Reid. He was on board with my mom coming because he knew we could use the extra moral support and because we were doing something different than the last two transfers. Reid wore a different shirt, which feels silly even to mention since the shirt he wore had absolutely nothing to do with whether this transfer would be successful. But that's how much we were clinging to faint hope. He had worn the same "Expect Miracles" shirt for the last two transfers, so he decided his Chicago Cubs shirt would do the trick this time. They had just won the World Series in 2016, so surely they'd bring us some luck. I still wore my Expect Miracles shirt but chose a different color. I think I had it in every color by this point, and it had become my daily uniform.

My doctor came into the pre-procedure area. As soon as he walked in, I said, "Did you see our surprise?"

He responded, "I did. We are transferring two embryos today? One of the abnormal ones, along with your untested embryo?"

I gave him a nervous smile and nodded my head. "Are we crazy?" I asked him.

He smiled and replied, "No, you're not crazy. But I want to make sure you understand the risks. This embryo could actually be trisomy 13. Not likely, but it's a possibility that I want to make sure you're aware of before we do this."

I knew from our research Trisomy 13 came with its own severe risks for the baby and me if that were the case. I looked at Reid and then my mom. Reid had no doubts. My mom gave me a knowing look to trust my gut. "Yes, we're okay with the risks," I told Dr. Griffith.

"Okay, then. Let's get you pregnant!" he said. He knew Reid and I were researchers, and we didn't make any decisions lightly. We knew he was in our corner and wanted to see us succeed in all areas of our lives.

We walked into the procedure room once again, and I climbed onto the table, putting my legs into stirrups. When I thought about starting a family at twenty-something, this was not how I imagined it - with a room full of people – my doctor, an embryologist, two nurses, my husband, and my mom. We all watched intently on the screen as the doctor took a catheter and placed our last two embryos in my uterus.

*Lord, please let this be it.*

We went home that afternoon, and I went to my "spot" on the couch to start my three days of bed rest. My mom made me a delicious soup because I had heard that keeping your belly warm helped implantation. I ate the warm soup, and with each bite, I prayed it would keep our embryos nice and warm in my uterus. *Please grow into healthy babies,* I prayed. We watched funny shows because laughter also supposedly helped. But let's be honest, laughter never hurts, and it gave me something to focus on.

I went in for bloodwork two days later to check my progesterone and testosterone levels, and everything looked good. I continued to have it checked every few days and tried my best to stay busy. My heart knew we'd be okay no matter the results. But I prayed so hard at least one of these babies would be in our arms in nine months.

On September 13th – one week from our embryo transfer – the fertility clinic called. My heart dropped when I saw the clinic's name on my phone. I had done bloodwork that morning, and I just *knew* my nurse was calling to tell me my hormone levels had dropped. When I answered, she said, "Abby? Hey, just a second… Dr. Griffith wants to speak with you." *Shit* (in fact, I'm pretty sure I said exactly that on the phone).

Dr. Griffith got on the phone and said, "Abby?"

"Yes…" I responded nervously.

He replied, *"Expect miracles!* Because you are PREGNANT!"

You could hear the smile in his voice, and he chuckled a little from excitement.

Chills covered my entire body. "Wait, really? The numbers look okay??" I guarded my heart, waiting for the bad news that was sure to follow.

He replied, "The numbers look more than okay. You are pregnant, and we just couldn't wait to tell you and Reid."

Every time I had been pregnant before, there had always been a "but" that followed. I fell silent, waiting for it, but there was no "but" this time.

He read all the numbers to me, and my hCG level was high for it only being one week since my transfer.

"Do you think both of them implanted?" I asked. My heart fluttered at the idea of twins, but then I thought, *Don't be silly, Abby. That's a long stretch.*

"It's possible, but we won't know for another week or two. We will continue with bloodwork and get you scheduled for an ultrasound soon. You're pregnant. This is happening. We're all so excited for you guys." I realized he had me on speakerphone, and my two favorite nurses were standing in his office with him. They were all so excited for us and congratulated me. The excitement in their voices radiated through the phone, and I felt them standing right there with me. I paced around my living room, unsure of what to do with my body, as I was so overcome with joy.

Dr. Griffith said he'd see me soon, and one of the nurses asked me to hang on the line so we could set up my next few appointments.

While talking with her, I heard the garage door open. Reid had just pulled in from work. I told her he had just gotten home and asked if she wanted to share the news with him. She was thrilled to do so.

I ran into the laundry room to greet him and put her on speakerphone. He walked in, surprised to see me standing there, and I said, "Hey, Jenny from our clinic is on the phone. She wants to tell you something."

She said, "Congratulations, Daddy! Y'all are PREGNANT!"

Reid's face lit up, and he gave me the biggest hug. As he pulled away, I could tell he was waiting for the "but," just like I had been. I told him, "Everything looks good. There's no reason to worry right now. We're really pregnant!" I could see the disbelief on his face. Jenny said she'd let us go, and I would see her in the clinic in a few days.

When we hung up with her, I told Reid where all my numbers were. He said, "Oh my gosh, we're having twins, aren't we?" as he nervously laughed.

"We're not sure yet," I told him, praying I could soon answer yes.

"Wow. I can't believe it. So, no reason to worry?" he said. He had been just as deeply affected as I had after all our previous losses.

"No reason to worry," I told him with the biggest grin on my face, and we hugged again.

After all we'd been through, hearing this amazing news almost didn't seem real. Regardless, we were elated and knew we needed to celebrate—today, we were pregnant.

We decided to go out to our favorite restaurant for dinner. But first, I had to make a few phone calls. I couldn't NOT share this amazing news with those closest to us. And if things did end up going south, I knew I would need them.

# Chapter 22

# Hope...Wait...Worry...Hope

## Fall 2018

The next few weeks were nerve-wracking, exciting, terrifying, and anxiety-ridden. I remember being filled with hope and excitement for our future, and then the next minute, I became crippled with fear of what could go wrong. With our history of pregnancy losses, fearing the worst had become the norm. Sometimes, it felt ridiculous to think things could go right for once. We were pregnant but also unsure of when/if Reid would get his transplant.

During an IVF pregnancy, they do multiple betas (pregnancy tests to check your hormone levels). We were scheduled for bloodwork every two days during the first week or two. I held my breath each time we waited for the results. At least it felt that way. Fortunately, my hormone levels came back better than expected each time.

After the third beta, my heart just knew this pregnancy would stick. This would be our baby/babies. We wouldn't know for another week or so whether I was carrying one or two, but after all the bad news I had been sharing with our support system, I couldn't wait to tell them we were pregnant.

We decided to share our news that night via a video on our Facebook and Instagram accounts, which were dedicated to our journey with infertility and Reid's need for a liver transplant.

Filled with excitement and nerves, we sat next to each other at our kitchen table, my laptop in front of us, and shared the amazing news that we were pregnant. We knew we were taking a risk by sharing the news so early and so broadly, but since we had been open about everything during our journey, we wanted to let everyone in on our miracle. If something were to happen with the pregnancy, we would lean on the same support system for help through it.

We went in for our first ultrasound with this pregnancy the following week. Reid went with me, as we had both agreed I wouldn't be going to any of these ultrasounds alone. Discovering the loss of our second baby alone two years prior left me deeply traumatized.

I was five weeks and three days pregnant for this ultrasound. We saw one gestational sac with a fetal pole (one of the first developmental stages for an embryo during pregnancy) and what could be another gestational sac, but there wasn't a fetal pole present. We knew we had one baby growing right on track, and we thanked the Lord for that. Time would tell whether we had a second baby growing.

⸻

Our first potential living donor arrived in Cleveland that afternoon. Desmond got settled in and prepared for the two days of testing ahead of him. It felt incredibly surreal to have someone travel to a completely different state to sit in a hospital and undergo an array of tests to see if he may be the match that my husband needed.

I had a hard time not being at the hospital to support our friend, but I knew we'd need to get used to it since we might have to test multiple people before finding a match.

The next morning, I received a picture from Desmond showing he had just completed his bloodwork and was heading to the next appointment on his schedule. I appreciated that he kept me updated each step of the way. Reid and I felt completely overcome with gratitude for him for taking such a giant leap and spending the time to see if he was a match.

Later that afternoon, I headed to my acupuncture appointment. I had been going to the same acupuncture clinic but switched to a different location closer to home. I knew my childhood friend Amanda had an appointment right after me, so we made plans to catch up in between.

I shared the wonderful news of our pregnancy with my acupuncturist, Jamie, and told her everything looked great. She knew the difficult journey we had been through to get pregnant, and her excitement for our news became evident by the tears in her eyes.

We chatted, and then she started my treatment, placing needles all over my body. I had grown to appreciate this time, allowing me just to be. After the needles were in place, she turned on relaxing music and left the room for about 20 minutes.

I lay on the table, a feeling of peace washing over my entire body. We were pregnant, and our first potential living donor had almost completed his testing to see if he could be Reid's lifesaving match. We were moving forward and looking at a bright future.

As soon as the appointment ended, I stopped by the bathroom. I felt a little crampy but knew that could happen early in a pregnancy. I looked into the toilet to find a huge gush of blood. My heart sank into my stomach as I tried to catch my breath. Panic set in. I placed my hands over my face and my elbows on my knees as tears started falling.

*How could this be happening? What do I do to stop it?*

The cramps became more intense as I sat in the bathroom stall, shaking and trying to keep myself from screaming. I found a pad in my purse and put it in my underwear.

I looked at my watch.

It was 3:30, and I needed to get to my fertility clinic before they closed. I had to know what was going on – stat.

My gut felt it already knew.

I rushed out of the bathroom and almost collided with Amanda as she walked toward the acupuncture clinic. She greeted me with a huge smile and a hug. I began sobbing again as she wrapped her arms around me.

She pulled away to look at me. "What's wrong?" she asked.

"I just had a huge gush of blood, and I'm cramping. I have no idea what's going on, but I can't lose this pregnancy. This can't be happening again."

Amanda pulled me back in for a tight hug as more tears escaped. She agreed I needed to get to the fertility clinic, so she told me to go quickly but to take deep breaths. "Please keep me updated," she said, "I will be praying so hard." I thanked her and walked out of that building as fast as possible. Each minute counted, and it would take me at least 20 minutes to get to the clinic.

When I got in the car, I called my nurse at the fertility clinic. The tone of her voice told me she knew this couldn't be good, but she tried to remain positive. She knew all the trauma we had been through and heard the panic in my voice. She instructed me to come straight in and assured me we would figure it out once I arrived. My doctor wasn't there, but another doctor could do the ultrasound.

I had texted Reid from the bathroom, and he left work early to meet me at the clinic. I called him after I got off the phone with the nurse, and I could tell the worry had also set in for him. We were both so afraid we might be losing the baby/babies.

Reid would likely beat me to the clinic. "I will wait in the parking lot for you. Please breathe… we don't know anything yet," he tried to reassure me, but I could hear he was also terrified. My fears consumed me, and it felt ignorant of me to believe things could be okay after the amount of blood I just saw.

My cramps became more intense as I drove to the clinic. I just knew I was miscarrying, and there was nothing I could do to stop it. My heart ached as I envisioned it being ripped out of my chest once again.

I later learned that Reid spent his entire drive to the clinic blaming himself for this. He had been so adamant about transferring the mosaic embryo, and now he worried we would have another pregnancy loss as a result.

I pulled into the hospital's parking lot and parked next to Reid. We shared a quick hug and then darted inside, begging for answers. The receptionist assured me my nurse would be right out.

She came out, hugged me, and said they would do the ultrasound first and bloodwork next. I walked into the exam room, removed my pants and underwear, and began to cry again as I saw the amount of blood I had lost during the drive to the clinic. I climbed onto the exam table and placed a sheet over my lap, waiting for the nurse and doctor.

"I just don't see how we can get good news out of this," I told Reid as we waited. My body shivered with panic as tears streamed down my cheeks.

Dr. Sorkin entered and asked me what happened. I told him about the bleeding and cramping, which seemed to be getting worse steadily. He said we'd talk more after the ultrasound, but he didn't want to waste any time because he knew we were eager to see what was happening.

He pulled up the ultrasound and turned the monitor to us. A heartbeat—a clear heartbeat. They usually didn't see a heartbeat that early in a pregnancy, but we saw it—beating away. And then we saw another very clear gestational sac with a fetal pole.

In the 30 hours since our last ultrasound, both babies had grown significantly, and the ultrasound confirmed I was carrying twins.

Reid and I both burst into tears… just seeing a heartbeat had us emotional, but now we knew we were pregnant with twins.

Dr. Sorkin searched all over my uterus to find the source of the bleeding, but everything looked perfectly fine.

Once we were done with the ultrasound, he asked what medications I was taking and when I took them. He also asked if anything else had been different. This time, they had put me on Lovenox, a blood thinner, which my doctor thought we would try to see if it helped.

Dr. Sorkin thought the Lovenox could be the culprit of the bleeding and said he would talk to Dr. Griffith to make sure he was okay with me stopping that medication. He assured us everything looked great from what he saw. He wanted me to have bloodwork and come back in two days to make sure the babies continued to grow, but the bleeding and cramping did not concern him.

I let out a huge breath and felt the tension release from every part of my body. I walked into the clinic that day so sure I was miscarrying, and I walked out knowing we were having twins. Talk about a roller coaster ride.

After the bloodwork draw, I got hugs from my favorite nurses, and Reid and I headed home. They put me on bed rest for a few days just to be safe, and I gladly accepted, knowing what the alternative could have been. My nerves were completely shot from the whirlwind of those last few hours, so putting on pajamas and sprawling on the couch sounded perfect.

The clinic followed up with us, letting me know Dr. Griffith approved me to stop taking Lovenox and agreed it may have caused the extra bleeding. Thankfully, he wasn't concerned. They also increased my nightly PIO (progesterone in oil) injection to 3 ml.

Two days later, we heard two beautiful heartbeats. Things were right on track. *This was really happening.*

---

Desmond finished his testing in Cleveland, and we were awaiting the results. They suspected his liver may not be the right fit for Reid, but we had to wait for some additional test results to come back. His case also had to be reviewed by their team of doctors to confirm.

---

The weeks following were filled with anticipation and anxiety. I continued to have spotting, but the doctor assured me that was normal as we watched the babies grow right on track through many ultrasounds. I had all-day sickness (why do they call it morning sickness? It's rarely just in the mornings), and there were very few things I could eat.

The wait to see if Desmond was a match continued, and the next appointment to see the babies and ensure they were growing on track was right around the corner.

Each time we passed a milestone that proved the babies were growing as they should, we breathed a huge sigh of relief. We made it past the point where we lost our previous pregnancies, and our NIPT testing came back clear at ten weeks. We felt we might finally become parents – to *twins*.

We learned Desmond wasn't going to be the match we needed, which broke our hearts, but we also knew going into this process, we may have to test several people before finding a match.

My best friend's brother had reached out and wanted to be tested, so he and his wife flew to Cleveland a few weeks later. He went through all the testing and became a potential match, but they needed a little more time for him to be healthy enough for the donation. When he called to tell me, he already had a plan and timeline to make the necessary changes to move forward with the process. The sacrifices other people were making for us continued to amaze me.

Reid and I agreed we needed to continue testing others in the meantime. We were very fortunate to have a list of people who had come forward, and we started the process of having another friend of mine from high school tested.

As my belly grew and we passed each milestone with the twins, we felt the stakes increased. Our friends and family constantly asked for updates because they also felt the pressure and were praying hard for Reid to have his liver transplant before the babies were born. Healthy babies, healthy daddy – that was the goal.

Reid and I figured with the way things were going, he would be in Cleveland receiving a living donor liver at the same time I would be giving birth to our twins in Houston. It would be excruciating for us not to be together for those monumental events, but it hardly felt fair to complain as that would mean we were getting everything we had prayed for. We had contingency plans for all scenarios and did our best to remain positive that everything would work out. I kept telling people, "I have no idea what the next 6-7 months will bring, but I'm sure we are in for a wild ride."

# Chapter 23

## The Power of Social Media

### January 2019

The holidays hit a little differently in 2018. We were thrilled about what lay ahead for us. This was a huge improvement from the last couple of years when the holidays reminded us of our empty arms and the uncertainty of Reid's health. That uncertainty still lingered, but we felt like we were closer to him receiving a transplant.

Things were progressing well with the pregnancy, and we'd reached a point where we felt confident that we'd have our healthy babies in our arms in several months. The big question—would Reid be there for the birth of our twins? I had to believe he would be.

My mom called on January 12th while Reid and I were getting dressed for a friend's wedding reception. I sensed a different tone in her voice.

She confessed, "Abby, I really don't know what I've done, but I think there may be a potential directed donation for Reid."

My mom is one of those people who will go above and beyond for others, and she was absolutely in this fight with us. She told me more than once that we could not afford to lose hope. Her insistent optimism shone through in difficult moments, as she often reassured me that everything would be okay. I appreciated her outlook, but after all we'd been through, I struggled to follow such optimism.

My mom wanted so badly to trust that Reid would get a directed liver donation, but I only saw the far-fetched side of it. I'm the realist who lived this journey so far, and we had already had two potential directed donations fall through.

My mom explained that a friend of hers sent her a Facebook message. She had seen a post by another mutual friend's friend whose son had just been in a tragic skiing accident in Colorado. The son, Clayton Sparks, had critical brain injuries, and they were keeping him on life support long enough to donate his organs, as they knew this was something he felt passionate about.

My mom contacted the mutual friend, Jackie, and asked if she thought Clayton's family would be open to discussing directed donation. She knew they were dealing with a tremendous loss and didn't want to be insensitive to that, but she also had a gut feeling this could be the life-saving match her son-in-law needed.

Jackie expressed her admiration for the family and knew they were kind people who would want to help another family in this way. Hearing that propelled my mom into action.

My mom then went back to Facebook, commented on the original post, and expressed her sincere sadness for the family. She followed with a gentle mention that her son-in-law was waiting for a liver in Houston if they would consider a directed donation. What an ask.

How might a question like that be taken during the worst moments of their life? My mom's determination to see her son-in-law be an active, healthy father to the twins growing inside her daughter allowed her to put it out there. These babies were a miracle for which she prayed hard; if God was willing, she wanted one more miracle.

At that same moment, Beth Sparks, Clayton's mom, was on the phone with her sister, who had Beth's Facebook post open in front of her. She saw my mom's comment and read it to Beth. Right away, Beth said, "I've got to go. I need to talk to our doctor and see if we can make this happen."

Without hesitation, amid immeasurable grief, Beth Sparks reached out to my mom to gather all of the information needed to save my husband's life. She then went to Clayton's doctor and told him they wanted to make a directed donation to Reid.

The doctor told Beth they would try, but he had never seen a successful directed donation. He actually told her, "There is a one-in-a-million chance this will work, but we will try."

Beth *believed* it would work. She messaged my mom and told her what the doctor had said and that she would keep her posted if she learned anything else.

Beth and her husband, Larry, then went to our Facebook page and learned more about us, our journey through infertility, and the fight for a liver transplant. Discovering that I grew up only 20 minutes from where Clayton did, and our families lived only 40 minutes away filled them with hope that they could witness first-hand how their son saved someone else's life.

Reid and I were unaware of what had been transpiring. We knew my mom had reached out and were hopeful, but we knew it would be a long shot. We went to our friend's wedding reception, knowing that if it did indeed work out, we weren't far from home and could get back to the hospital if needed.

Clayton's doctor came to Beth that evening and told her the directed donation might be a match. They were moving forward with

Clayton's liver being directed to Reid. Beth then messaged my mom to share the latest update.

In the middle of the wedding reception, my mom called me. She uttered through tears, "Abby, I think this may happen. He's a blood type match, and it looks like everything is lined up for them to make a directed donation." I looked at Reid as the tears started streaming down my face. I didn't have to say anything; he knew this long shot had become a strong possibility.

After I got off the phone with my mom, Reid and I agreed to head home and call the transplant center. We went to tell our friend we were leaving, and I shared that we may have a potential liver offer. She began crying and said she would be praying for us.

When we got in the car, I called our transplant center. It was a Saturday night, so I knew I would get whichever transplant coordinator was on call.

When the coordinator answered the phone, I explained why I was calling. She said, "Abby, I know exactly who you are and was just about to call you guys. We are still checking a few things, but it seems this liver is a good match for your husband."

I went quiet as I tried to hold back the tears, wrapping my free arm around my pregnant belly. I told Jaymee, the coordinator, "I'm pregnant with twins, and we've been so afraid my husband wouldn't get his transplant before our babies arrive." I gasped for breath as tears escaped.

She responded, "Oh my gosh, now I'm going to cry."

Jaymee told us to go home and eat a late dinner, and then Reid shouldn't have anything to eat or drink after midnight. She didn't know what time the surgery would be or when we'd get called to the hospital, but all signs pointed to this being the match he needed. She told us to try to get some rest and wait for a call early the next morning.

As soon as I got off the phone with her, I called Reid's mom. Through a flood of tears, I told her he was likely going to have his transplant the following day. Next, I called my mom with the details and then the rest of our family and close friends who needed to know.

I remember riding home that night feeling surreal, like we were floating in a dream. I had been so afraid *the call* would never come, but now we were told Reid's lifesaving transplant would likely happen the next morning.

Once we got home, I decided to go Live on Facebook to share the news. We needed every person praying, not only for this to be the match for Reid but also for the donor's family and friends.

Reid went into the bedroom to pack his hospital bag, and I sat down on the couch, still in my dress from the wedding reception. My trembling fingers pushed the live button on Facebook. I took deep breaths, and my heart pounded as I saw people jumping on to watch the video. I shared that a family was directly donating a liver to Reid. My emotions kicked into overdrive during that live announcement. I was thrilled Reid might finally be getting a liver transplant the next day, but I had also learned more about the donor and his family, and my heart ached so badly for them.

Clayton, our donor, grew up just two small towns over from where I did. I later discovered that I babysat one of his college roommates when I was younger. Clayton was only 24 at the time of his accident. We knew so many of the same people, and the news of his death rocked the small town he grew up in.

I hadn't spoken directly with his parents, so I didn't reveal any information about the donor just yet.

I shared how excited we were to be preparing for a transplant, but I also reminded everyone watching that we could get to the hospital the next day and learn the liver wasn't a match for Reid. There were a lot of things that could happen between then and the transplant, and I was trying to manage not only our expectations but the expectations of others.

I then asked for prayers for the donor family. My whole body shook as I thought about them sitting in a hospital room signing paperwork to donate their son's organs to others.

They were saying their final goodbyes as we prepared for a new start.

I cried sharing the news because I felt so guilty for even being excited about what this meant for us. How in the world could we be happy knowing someone else was losing their son, friend, nephew, grandson, or boyfriend?

Once I finished the live video, I set my phone down and let the floodgates open.

We had been through four transplant education classes at different transplant centers. Still, nothing could have properly prepared me for the intense flood of emotions when we finally received that call, especially from a deceased donor's family.

The fact that we knew some of Clayton's family and friends intensified those feelings. In some way, it gave me comfort knowing we could have a relationship with them after the transplant, and they could see Clayton living on and even watch Reid become a dad. But at the same time, we were grieving the loss of a person we had never met.

I once again wrapped my arms around my belly and prayed we would never be in the position the Sparks family found themselves in that night.

While we mourned with them, I also knew we had to celebrate what this meant for us and truly recognize the life that was being given to my husband. Right then, I decided to do all I could to honor this amazing gift, regardless of whether this was the match Reid needed.

Reid came and sat with me on the couch for a bit, and we honestly didn't know what to say to each other. We switched to action mode and worked on the list of items Reid needed to pack. Then, we discussed plans for who would care for our dog.

We reminded each other of the possibility of this not happening and that we needed to set our expectations accordingly. We had heard of others getting called in multiple times for a transplant, and then additional testing would rule out the organ for them. We had to be realistic about it. I don't think either of us allowed ourselves to truly believe it was happening until they wheeled him back to surgery. And even then, plans could change.

We both had a late dinner and got ready for bed. Somehow, we needed to get a few hours of sleep, even though our adrenaline would likely make that impossible.

As we lay in bed, I tried to respond to the flood of messages and social media comments that had already come in. Our support system showed they were in this with us, for which we were so grateful.

Reid and I both turned up the volume on our phones and tried to sleep. I'm pretty sure neither of us got more than two hours of sleep that night. We each kept waking up to check our phones, anticipating heading to the hospital at any moment.

The next morning, around 8 AM, I texted Jaymee. She said the donor's surgery needed to be scheduled before we would have an OR (operating room) time, and that hadn't happened yet. She told us to expect a call in the next hour or two, but the surgery likely wouldn't happen until later that evening.

Around 10 AM, we got the call to grab our bags and head to the transplant center.

# Chapter 24

## Waiting for Clayton's Final Gift

### January 13–14, 2019

We loaded our bags in the car and headed to the Texas Medical Center.

I called and texted a few of our family and friends to let them know we were on our way. One of those calls was to Denise. Reid wanted me to have her there for all of it. His parents would be there, of course, but he was their son, and they would be worried about *him* (as they should be). Reid wanted one person there to care for *me* (and our babies) throughout this.

He knew the emotional stress of the transplant would be extremely tough on me.

When we called Denise from the car, we had her on speakerphone. Reid told her he wanted her to ensure I ate, drank plenty of water, and rested when I could. "I'm on it," she replied. We knew we could count on my bossy best friend.

I asked her to give us a little time before heading to the hospital. I knew we had a long road ahead of us, and today would include a lot of sitting and waiting.

My mom would have been there with me, but she had to be at a different hospital that day, an hour and a half away, prepping for my stepdad's back surgery the following day. She said she would drive to Houston once we got settled in, but I worried about her making the drive. Plus, we didn't even know if this liver would work out yet, so I told her not to come.

I know it was hard for her to not be there in person. If the surgery did happen, it would likely be in the very early morning hours, and I didn't see how my mom could be there for us and make it back in time for my stepdad's surgery.

Once we arrived at the hospital, we confidently made our way to Reid's hospital room on the transplant floor. We felt comfortable knowing the entire floor was dedicated to transplant patients. That meant everyone we came into contact with would be familiar with the process we were (hopefully) about to go through.

Our nurse checked us into the room, and then, after we chatted, she walked over to the whiteboard and wrote down her name and Reid's preferred name. Then she wrote "Happy Liver Day!" and drew a big smiley face. Goosebumps covered my arms and legs as I read what she wrote.

As Reid's parents arrived, the transplant team came in to perform several tests. They needed to make sure nothing significant had changed in his health and his body could handle the intense surgery. The testing went well, and things continued to move forward. Every time someone from the medical team walked into Reid's hospital room, I sucked in air, and my entire body tensed. I kept expecting one of them to tell us this wouldn't work.

We had a visit with a member of the medical research team. He told us about an opportunity to sign up for a clinical trial they were doing. The trial would give Reid a 50/50 chance of having the donated liver placed on a perfusion machine during transport. They often do this for kidneys, but this was a relatively new concept for livers. The liver perfusion machine pumps oxygenated blood through the liver during transport, which, in theory, would not only allow the liver to survive outside of a human body for longer but also allow them to see how the organ worked to further determine suitability for transplantation.

Reid and I got excited about these types of medical advances, so we had no hesitations about participating in the trial. Reid signed the paperwork, and within a few minutes, the medical staff let us know we were selected for the study group and that the donor's liver would be on a perfusion machine during transport to Houston. Knowing this advanced procedure would be a part of the transplant journey reassured us that things were headed in the right direction.

That afternoon, Reid's transplant team came by to tell us our potential donor, Clayton, would be going into surgery at 9:30 that night. Therefore, three members of our transplant team would be flying to Colorado around 6 PM to be there for the surgery. They would evaluate the liver and potentially perform a biopsy on the organ to ensure compatibility for Reid. If they elected to do a biopsy right after they removed the liver, the team would have to wait there for the results, which would add an hour to their trip.

Assuming everything checked out after Clayton's surgery, we were told Reid's surgery was scheduled for 3 AM the next morning.

We settled into our hospital room and attempted to take a nap, praying so hard this transplant would be successful. Reid gave me the hospital bed so I could try to get some actual sleep, and he took the small couch in the room. His parents went down to the cafeteria to grab some dinner.

After our transplant team flew up to Colorado and Clayton had his surgery, they sent news back that the liver looked good, and they pushed Reid's surgery time to 4 AM since things took a bit longer than expected in Colorado. They decided not to do a biopsy on the liver, which we took as a good sign.

When Denise arrived at the hospital around 2 AM, she brought a massive bag of snacks, a pillow, and a blanket. Knowing I had someone there for *me* eased my mind so I could be there for my husband through all this.

This was happening.

I still tried to mentally prepare myself while keeping my heart guarded. Reid could go into surgery, and the transplant team could decide the liver wasn't perfect for him. But we had an OR time, and our team was heading back to Houston with the liver for my husband.

A little before 4 AM, they came to take Reid down for his surgery. As they wheeled him out, Denise asked if we could pray over Reid before he went down. We stood in the hallway of the transplant floor with our heads bowed. Denise prayed for the surgeons and the team involved in Reid's surgery, and she prayed for the Sparks family. She lived in the same small town that Beth and Larry Sparks did, so she saw first-hand the tremendous loss in this community—that moment of prayer calmed my inner anxieties.

They wheeled Reid down to the pre-op area as we followed. We stood in the hallway talking with the anesthesiologist, then said our goodbyes as they took my husband back into the surgical area. We learned the team wasn't back with the liver yet, but they expected them shortly and would let us know when the surgery started. In the meantime, they prepped Reid for surgery.

We entrusted Reid to the care of those dedicated to saving his life, and a nurse showed us to the family waiting room. The nurse said she would be in the surgery with Reid and would be the one to update us. This relieved me as I sensed she truly cared about the surgery's success. It put me at ease knowing she would be at his side, taking care of him.

The waiting room was completely empty at that early morning hour. The hospital volunteer who manned the waiting room desk had not even arrived for the day's shift. My mind and body were physically exhausted already but fueled by adrenaline.

Denise did her job as my wellness coach and reminded me often to eat. She kept walking to the water station down the hall to refill my 32-ounce cup with water.

There were only chairs in the waiting room, so we moved some around to make a makeshift couch so I could lie down. I knew I needed to take care of myself and our babies through this process as well… labor at 21 weeks was the last thing we needed right now. But I also trusted that our babies were tough and we had gotten this far. We would all be okay, one way or another.

Reid's parents walked to the hotel across the street from the hospital and checked into a room. They planned to nap a little since he was back in surgery, or so we thought. We were prepared for the long process ahead but exhausted from the stress of the last 36 hours. And the transplant hadn't even officially started yet.

About an hour after Reid went back to the pre-op area, our nurse came to provide an update. She said the liver and team hadn't arrived yet, but they hoped to start his anesthesia and open him up soon. The prep team would have him ready so that when the liver did arrive, the transplant team could get right to work. Their estimated arrival time was 6 AM, so I laid down and attempted to nap without much success.

An hour passed, and the nurse came out again to share they had just put him under anesthesia and were opening up his abdomen to prepare for surgery. In a few hours, she would be back to give me an update.

I settled in for a nap since surgery seemed to be starting, and we wouldn't get another update for a while.

# Chapter 25

# Of Course, It Couldn't Be Easy

## January 14, 2019

I had finally nodded off to sleep on my uncomfortable but adequate makeshift couch in the waiting room.

"Abby... Abby, wake up," Denise said as she patted my leg. Three surgeons had just walked into the waiting room and asked the hospital volunteer for the family of Timothy (Reid) Gray. Denise overheard them and woke me up as they headed towards us.

I had no idea what time it was or how much time had passed. I quickly asked Denise the time as I tried to wake myself up enough to have whatever conversation they were coming here for. "Almost 8 AM," she said. *This can't be good.*

The lead surgeon, Dr. Gohar, asked if we could move to the tables in the corner of the room to talk. He looked down at my pregnant belly as I stood up to join them. I could see in his face that he was not ready to deliver whatever news he had for me.

We sat down, and I studied the faces of the three surgeons, pleading with my eyes for everything to be okay. Dr. Gohar said that Reid was open on the table and under anesthesia, but they needed *me* to decide whether or not to move forward with the surgery.

The liver had been in transit for longer than they anticipated. Having it transported on the perfusion machine helped, but there wasn't enough evidence to prove it could sustain livers as long as this one had been on the machine. Because of the extra risks, they could not decide to move forward with the surgery; I had to be the one to make that call.

I sat in front of three very stoic surgeons as they asked me to make a life-altering decision.

Do we move forward with this transplant and assume the risk that his body may reject the liver? Or do they close him back up, and then I have to tell my husband I chose not to move forward with the surgery, putting him back in the same spot we were a few days ago?

Dr. Gohar went on to explain the very serious dangers associated with moving forward with the surgery, which is why they could not make the decision. They could lose him on the table when they placed the liver in his abdomen. The liver could cause his body to shut down, affecting his other organs as well. His body may be more likely to reject the liver, which would then land him in the ICU until they could hopefully find another liver to save him.

But if this worked, it would completely change our world and save my husband's life.

My eyes swelled as I tried to remain calm and consider the options. I asked Denise to call Reid's parents and have them return immediately. They needed to be a part of this conversation as well.

I sat for a minute and then asked Dr. Gohar, "If this were your son, what would you do?" His body tensed, and he looked at me with teary eyes.

He replied, "Abby, I can't make that decision for you. All I can do is give you the risks and allow you to determine what we do next."

I searched the faces of the other surgeons again, hoping one of them would give me some sign that it was okay to move forward. They all sat there with tears in their eyes, and I could feel their sympathy for our situation. I explained to them that Dr. Raijman truly believed Reid had cholangiocarcinoma, but we couldn't find it. I further explained my worries that if I didn't move forward with this, I would lose him to cancer before he was able to get a liver transplant.

I wrapped my arms around my belly.

Not only did I have the fate of my *husband* in my hands, but he was also the *father of our unborn twins,* and the outcome would directly affect all three of us.

Without a doubt, I knew the decision Reid would make if he were sitting here right now, but I also knew I couldn't lose him. The pain of making this decision, one that could potentially end his life on the operating table that day, ripped through me like a category-five hurricane. I knew what I had to do, but I needed some reassurance.

Denise looked at me and said, "Abby, Reid's parents are coming. But you need to know what you want to do before they arrive. You know what Reid would want, and you know what you feel is best. As his wife, you are the one who has to make the decision." Tears streamed down her face as she encouraged me to follow my heart. She would not give her opinion one way or the other, but she let me know she had the utmost confidence in my ability to make this decision.

I looked at the surgeons and said, "We're moving forward with the surgery." As those words came out, I focused on their faces for a reaction. They gave none. I'm not sure if I imagined it, but I *felt* a sense of relief from them.

This surgical team had Reid's life in their hands as I asked them to move forward with the risky surgery. My heart told me I could trust them to take the responsibility seriously.

I requested they also discuss this with Reid's parents. I needed his parents to be able to ask questions of the surgical team, even though the decision had been made. I prayed they would feel the same way I did.

Ric and Tinker emerged into the waiting room out of breath. Their faces were pale and distraught as they beelined towards the tables where we sat. It was apparent they had run from the hotel after receiving Denise's call. I looked at Dr. Gohar and asked him to share the same information he had shared with us.

I watched as Tinker searched their faces just as I had. She then looked at me as tears slid down her cheeks. I told her I felt confident that if Reid were sitting here right now, he would say to move forward with the surgery. There wasn't a fiber in my body that doubted it.

She looked at Dr. Gohar and asked the same question I did: "If it were your son, what would you do?" I knew he wanted so badly to answer the question honestly as he watched tears fall down Tinker's and Ric's faces. But his answer remained the same as it had been for me. He couldn't make that decision for us.

Tinker went on to ask more pointed medical questions, and she and Ric came to the same conclusion I had – we had to take the risk.

We all agreed we were moving forward with the surgery, and the three surgeons stood to return to the operating room. They assured us our nurse would give updates as often as she could and that the surgery would likely take 6-8 hours. They would do all they could to save my husband; I had no reservations about it.

After they left the waiting room, a moment of panic set in. *What if I had just made a decision that would ultimately take my husband's life?* I tried not to let my fear show, as I didn't want his parents worrying the same (as if they weren't already).

*If the worst were to happen, would they blame me for the rest of their lives?* I knew I would certainly blame myself. I held my breath, praying Reid would be okay. I sat there attempting to hide my emotions from everyone around me as the waiting room started to fill with other families waiting for their loved ones.

My dad and step-mom stopped by, and it meant so much that they made the trip there; I knew how hard it was for my dad to be in a hospital after the death of his mom a few years prior. I wanted to express my gratitude for them being there, but I barely had the words to form a sentence. I mostly sat in silence as the others tried their best to small-talk.

Then, a couple of hospital volunteers walked in with emotional support dogs. I choked back tears and felt this was a sign that my husband would be okay. If Reid were sitting in this waiting room at that moment, he would be overjoyed to see these dogs.

It hit me then how much we had been through **together**. My husband was currently lying open on an operating table, and I did not have him there to process my feelings with me. But I knew I couldn't get caught up in those emotions. I had to keep my feelings to myself right then because I was afraid that if I opened the floodgates, I wouldn't be able to shut them again.

As the dogs walked over to where we were sitting, I bent down to pet one, and a few tears slipped out. I wiped them away quickly, feeling silly for crying about seeing dogs. I'm not even the big dog lover; Reid is.

I sucked in a breath and told Denise and Reid's parents that maybe it was time for me to go take a nap in the hotel room.

Reid was well into his surgery by then and would be for a while. The tough decision had been made, and whatever came next would come, whether I was there in the waiting room or napping in the hotel room. But I still struggled to leave the hospital. Reid's parents encouraged me to go rest and said they would be there for updates and would let me know.

Denise and I walked over to the hotel. I propped three pillows against the headboard of the bed and tried to do some deep breathing to calm my anxiety. Denise had asked Tinker to update us via her phone so I could sleep. She turned up the volume on her phone and then laid down to nap.

My phone had many unread messages, social media posts, and missed calls. I had tried to keep up with the messages and respond to everyone, but I felt completely overwhelmed. I just couldn't.

Knowing we had such a huge support group behind us had always eased my mind, but I also felt I needed to express our appreciation to each person who reached out. At that point, though, I barely had the capacity to form a thought. I turned off all social media notifications and let the texts go unread for now.

I needed to quiet my mind and body for an hour or two. I had to remember the two tiny lives growing inside me were also my responsibility, and I needed to take care of them during this difficult time.

When I woke up from my nap, Denise had news for me. I could tell she had been up a little longer than I had, and I sensed her worry. She knew I was exhausted and could not change the situation, so she let me sleep.

She told me Reid's parents had called a bit ago, and he had experienced some complications during the surgery. When they went to put the new liver in, his entire system started shutting down. They managed to stabilize him, but it took quite a while. They planned to get to a point where they could finish up for the day, and then they would resume the surgery the next day. They still had another hour or two to go, so there wasn't a rush to get back right now.

I took a quick shower and changed my clothes, and then Denise and I walked back to the hospital.

Reid's mom looked worried, but I could also tell she was attempting to put on a brave face when I walked in. They said the surgery should be wrapping up soon, and the nurse would come back out to let us know.

We sat in the waiting room and tried to keep it light-hearted. As of right then, Reid was okay. We just needed him to get through the night, undergo another surgery, and be on the road to recovery. Several friends and family stopped by the hospital that day with food, coffee, and emotional support.

As alone as I felt not having Reid sitting by my side, I felt surrounded by many others who loved us and were here on this journey—whether in person or spirit.

I asked Reid's mom for more information about the latest update from the surgery. Then I decided to reach out to some trusted resources for more information and, hopefully, reassurance that he would be okay. I had made a few connections through social media with others who had either been through this process with their loved ones or were in the medical field helping transplant patients.

I contacted them to let them know the situation, and they reassured me that the team finishing the surgery the next day was not completely unheard of. His body needed to rest after the stress of the transplant, and reconnecting his bile ducts (the last step of the surgery) could wait. Hearing that provided so much comfort.

That afternoon, around 3 PM, I got a call from our transplant coordinator, Vita, whom we had grown to know well. She said Reid was out of surgery and in the ICU. I could come back to see him, but she wanted to let me know they had placed him back on the transplant list.

When a transplant patient has their surgery, they are removed from the list. But now she told me the team added Reid back on the list. That couldn't be good.

"This is purely a precaution," she said. "Hopefully, his body will start accepting the liver soon." They were concerned with how his body reacted when they placed the liver inside, so they wanted to be extra vigilant and make sure we were all prepared in case he started to go into rejection.

She said two people at a time were allowed to head to the ICU to see Reid when we were ready. I shared the update with everyone, and then Tinker and I headed back to see him.

When I walked in the double sterile doors to the ICU area, Vita stood just inside the door. I wrapped my arms around her and started sobbing. She assured me they would take care of my husband, and he was stable for now.

I thanked her for everything and headed back to Reid's room.

# Chapter 26

# Clayton's Gift, Humbly Received

### January 14-16, 2019

Nothing can ever fully prepare you for seeing the person you love most, your life partner, intubated in the ICU.

I entered the room to find Reid lying flat on his back. Machines beeped loudly all around him.

My heart raced as my eyes darted around at all of the cords and tubes coming out of him. He had a tube down his throat, which prevented his head from moving, and his eyes were open as we walked in. One large tube was coming out of the side of his neck, and he had several more tubes coming out of his abdomen and chest. He had a tiny tube taped to his nose that was going from his nose down into his stomach. His hands were secured to the bed frame with velcro straps to keep him from pulling out any of the tubes or IVs as the anesthesia wore off.

A lump formed in my throat as I forced myself not to break down in front of him. I knew it had to be hard on him to lay there, unable to speak or move. I refused to make it harder by having him worry about my emotional state.

I leaned over his bed and looked him in the eye. "Everything will be okay. The liver is in, but they'll finish connecting the bile ducts tomorrow." I searched his face for understanding and tried to determine if he needed to know more. I knew not to give Reid the full details until he could ask questions. Recovery should be his main focus right now. I needed him to fight to stay alive for me and our babies.

He nodded very slightly, and I could see the pain in his eyes. I wondered if he could see the immense worry in mine.

A nephrologist (kidney doctor) walked into Reid's ICU room. "Mrs. Gray? May we speak outside for a moment?" *Shit.*

Once we were just outside the glass door to the ICU room, the nephrologist told me Reid's kidneys were reacting poorly to the transplant. They were considering placing him on dialysis.

The doctor had concerns and laid out their action plan. "We will see what his latest bloodwork says and decide based on that," he shared. They were trying to avoid his kidneys shutting down after all the stress his body had just been through.

As we wrapped up our conversation, a nurse approached the nephrologist and said Reid's kidney numbers were significantly improving. I could see the shock on the doctor's face, and he asked to see the results.

The nurse handed over his tablet, and he scanned the results, looked at me, and declared, "Good news, we don't need dialysis right now. We will continue to monitor him, but if his numbers keep improving like this, his kidneys should be fine." My sigh of relief echoed against the glass door separating me and my husband.

Visiting hours were now over, so I went back in to tell Reid we would return in a few hours when they allowed visitors again. "Try to rest," I told him. "If the nurses or doctors need to call me, they will."

I walked out of his ICU room and broke down as I slid the door to his room shut. I never imagined how hard it would be to see him like that. And even if I had, he looked much worse than I could have envisioned. He was my person. He would be optimistic in this situation and help me through it. But he couldn't even communicate with me.

A sweet nurse approached me and wrapped her arms around me as I tried to pull myself together. She heard about our story and had already taken the time to read a few of my blog posts about our journey to this day. She assured me they were doing everything possible and Reid was in the best hands. I'm not sure she'll ever know how much her compassion made a difference in that moment.

After leaving the ICU, we stopped by the family waiting room, where Denise and Ric were waiting. We had a few more hours until ICU visiting hours opened again, and it was now dinner time. Reid's parents decided I should stay at the hotel, and they would go home for the night to rest.

Denise and I walked back to the hotel room to try to relax for a little bit.

I called Beth Sparks, Clayton's mom, on our walk to the hotel. She had texted me earlier to check on Reid, and I wanted to finally talk to the person who made this incredible decision to save my husband's life.

Beth and Larry were home with a house full of Clayton's friends. Beth stepped into her bedroom to talk to me, and we instantly connected through all the emotions we were both feeling. I felt overcome with worry for my husband, and she was grieving the loss of her son.

She asked about Reid and the transplant, so I gave her an optimistic update. I did not want her to stress about him, and I felt an extra sense of responsibility now that Clayton's liver lived inside Reid's body. We all needed this to work. I did not want to have to tell her later that Reid's body had not accepted her son's liver.

Beth described Clayton's personality to me, but I already knew in my heart that he had lived a kind and generous life. We agreed to talk later, and I told her I would keep her posted on Reid's recovery and subsequent surgery.

My sister, Megan, met us at the hotel with dinner.

The moment we stepped into the hotel room, another overwhelming wave of emotion hit me. My whole body trembled as I sobbed uncontrollably. I collapsed on the bed and gasped for breath.

"I can't do this. I can't hold it together without him," I told Denise and Megan.

"You *can* do this. He isn't going anywhere. We aren't going anywhere either." Denise tried to reassure me.

Reid had been by my side through all the hard times, but he wasn't here now. We had no idea how the next 24 hours would go. He couldn't even communicate how he felt, and I couldn't tell him the whole story of what had happened that day.

I placed both hands on my belly as I lay in the fetal position, pleading for everything to be okay. They assured me that, no matter what, they were here and would see me through whatever happened next. The babies and I would be okay. Reid is strong, and he would fight to survive this.

After letting me have a full-on breakdown, Denise told me I needed to pull it together for my babies. We started deep breathing together, and my body slowly began to relax. I needed that release of emotions, but I had to pivot and focus on myself and our babies.

I couldn't do anything for Reid except allow the exceptional medical team to continue to care for him.

We settled in and enjoyed the dinner Megan brought us—fajitas and my comfort food, chips and queso. Shortly after we ate, I jumped on social media to give a live update on Reid. Once again, I gave the optimistic version but shared how hard it had been to see him in his current state.

I still couldn't read all the messages and social media posts on my phone, so I wanted to update everyone all at once instead of responding individually to each message.

After the update on social media, we turned on the local news. Beth had shared that one of the local stations had come to interview them that day about Clayton's accident and his choice to be an organ donor. As their story aired, Denise, Megan, and I watched in complete silence. Megan grabbed a box of tissues so we could wipe away the tears streaming down our faces. My heart beamed with pride that the Sparks family used this opportunity to spread the important message of organ donation and to share the legacy their son left behind.

A news reporter had reached out to me earlier that day, but with all the uncertainty after Reid's first surgery and the day's stress, I told them I would have to speak with them the next day. I wanted to share about the amazing gift we were being given, but I didn't feel I had the strength to do so yet.

The next morning, I awoke eager to see what the day held and how Reid had done through the night. At 5 AM, I headed back to the ICU during the first visitation time of the day.

Reid had done well overnight and was a little more alert, but they still had him fully intubated and on a lot of painkillers. He now had a letterboard to communicate with. He would point to each letter to spell whatever he wanted to say. It was nice to be able to communicate, but it also became frustrating for him, as he had blurry vision and unsteady hands.

He lifted his shaky hand as the monitors beeped all around him. I angled the letter board so he could see it from his stationary position in the bed. His hand moved slowly across the board; W-O-R-T-H-L-E-S-S. My heart sank as he looked at me, his eyes pleading to make it through this.

I asked, "Worthless?" He gently nodded his head as tears filled his eyes. I inquired, "Is that how you feel right now?" He softly nodded again.

He felt he couldn't do anything but lay there while everyone around him worried and cared for him. I knew he wanted to be able to communicate better with me and ask how I was handling it all. I reassured him, "I know it feels that way right now, but soon you will be better. We will get through this. I'm here and will be here through it all."

I later learned that at 2:00 that morning, before Reid had been given the letterboard, they told him they would be changing one of his medications. He wanted the team to run the medication change by me so I could ask questions first because he was nervous about his fragile condition. At that point, change was normal, but he needed me to advocate for him and be aware of the situation.

When the nurse told him about the change, he tried to signal him to call me. Reid kept pointing to where his wedding ring should be and then holding his hand in the shape of a phone to his ear. It took several tries before the nurse understood, and then he said, "Oh, you want me to call your wife? I can do that, but it's 2 AM." Reid immediately shook his head no. He had no concept of the time, and he knew I needed sleep with the events of the past couple of days. I honestly wished they had called and woke me to give him that extra peace of mind. I hated the thought of him lying there alone.

Ric and Tinker arrived back at the hospital early that morning.

Around 8 AM, they took Reid back for surgery to complete the transplant. At that point, they just needed to connect his bile ducts and properly close his abdomen. The team felt his body could withstand the final surgery now, and he seemed to be accepting his new liver.

Hearing that news released tension in my body that I didn't even realize I was holding onto.

*Lord, please let this mean everything is going to be okay.*

The transplant team worked tirelessly, continuously drawing blood and running tests to closely monitor his body's reaction to his new organ.

Ric and Tinker were visiting Reid in his ICU room shortly after the second surgery when one of the transplant surgeons came by with a group of medical students. She stood outside Reid's room, giving the students a run-down of Reid's last 36 hours. She told the students, "This case was scary. We nearly lost him on the table, and it took quite a while to get him stable again."

Tinker overheard this and could see in Reid's face that he also heard it. We had tried our best not to share how scary things had been the day before because we didn't want to worry Reid any more than he already was. Tinker immediately texted me to let me know what he heard, so I asked her to update him based on that information.

I hated that he had to hear how dire the situation had been when he couldn't ask the questions I knew he would have, but we also didn't want him lying there worrying.

Later that day, they extubated him. I felt so much better just being able to fully see my husband's face and talk with him. Reid's condition showed improvement, and he had made it through the first critical 24 hours with his "new" liver.

Reid slowly progressed over the next few days. Witnessing my husband, who had walked into the hospital just a few days before, now barely able to move, was excruciating.

Denise stayed with me for the first several days, and we made multiple trips back and forth from the hotel to the hospital daily during each of the ICU visiting hours. Each time I walked back and forth from the hospital to the hotel, my steps slowed as my belly felt heavier.

Reid's parents drove to the hospital each morning and stayed most of the day so they could also see him.

–––––––––––––––––––––––––––––––––––––––––––––––––––

Two days after the transplant, I had an appointment with my OB-GYN. I seriously debated rescheduling it because I had major anxiety about leaving the hospital. But everyone assured me I needed to go check on the babies, and Reid would be in good hands.

Denise drove me back to our side of town for my appointment. A friend who works with the medical team at my doctor's office had shared the news of Reid's transplant with them, so my doctor and the nurses asked how Reid was doing.

Then, my doctor talked with me about how *I* was doing and made sure I focused on myself and the babies during this time. He said, "I can't imagine the amount of stress you are feeling right now." As he spoke, I tried to relax, becoming aware that every muscle in my body felt tense.

They performed an ultrasound to check on the babies. We originally weren't scheduled for an ultrasound that day, but they added it, considering the tremendous stress I was under. It eased my anxiety to see our babies on the screen, squirming around with strong heartbeats.

We were 21 weeks and four days along in the pregnancy, but my belly measured 28 weeks at that appointment. It had grown significantly from the last week, and I could definitely feel the extra weight as the babies grew.

I knew my anxiety had skyrocketed with all we had been dealing with, and I tried my best to focus on what I could.

I don't think I fully understood the total weight of what we were going through until I was scrolling through Facebook on the way back to the hospital, and saw a post Denise's sister-in-law made on the day of Reid's transplant. I read it out loud to Denise as it sunk in. Her post said, "Next time I'm stressed, I'm going to remember that I'm not 'pregnant with miracle twins while husband has liver transplant' stressed. Some women are damn WARRIORS! **#abbylieveinmiracles**." It was both the comedic relief and reality check I needed.

# Chapter 27

## Complications

### January-February 2019

Three days after Reid's transplant, the team had him up and (very slowly) walking the halls of the ICU floor. His recovery progressed as well as they had hoped, and his body seemed to be accepting Clayton's liver. Reid's nutrients were received from the NG tube that went into his nose and down to his stomach.

Megan had a doctor's appointment that same day. We found out a month earlier she was pregnant (after her first month of trying - that bitch!), and she had her first ultrasound scheduled. We were between the ICU's visiting hours, so Denise, Ric, Tinker, and I were all downstairs getting lunch in the hospital cafeteria. After her appointment, my sister called and said, "Abby, you're not going to believe this… we're having twins."

I let out a laugh loud enough to get the attention of a few passersby. "No way. You're joking." I insisted.

She replied, "I know better than to joke with you about something like that right now. We are seriously having twins." After years of heartbreak and wondering whether Reid and I would ever have kids, my sister and I were now expecting twins *together*.

Joy flooded my body, and I couldn't believe what I had just heard. I couldn't wait to return to the ICU room and share the news with Reid.

As expected, hearing that my sister and her husband were also having twins brought Reid a big smile. "I told you!" he said. He had previously joked about how wild it would be if they were also to have twins.

Right after the twin excitement, Clayton's friends sent me a video. They were all sitting in the living room of Clayton's parents' house, sending their well wishes to Reid to let us know they were all in this with us.

Reid and I sat on the edge of his hospital bed together, and I held my phone in front of us. We both watched intently as these strangers showed such compassion during their time of great loss. They wanted so badly for Reid's body to accept Clayton's liver so they could watch him live on through another person.

Their kindness and support brought tears to our eyes, and we were both covered in goosebumps as we finished the video.

Later that night, they moved Reid out of ICU and to a recovery room on the transplant floor. His NG tube had been removed, so he progressed to a liquid diet. His pain levels were still high, but all his numbers seemed to be improving with each blood draw. The transplant team changed his bloodwork from every four hours to every eight hours.

The hospital staff at the transplant center went above and beyond to be helpful. When I said I would be staying in Reid's room with him, they made sure to have a recliner for me to sleep in. My stomach felt like I was carrying around a bowling ball at this point, so I could not sleep flat anymore, but I was absolutely not going home and leaving my husband alone in the hospital.

Even though Reid could talk and had been cleared to get up and use the bathroom alone, he was unquestionably not himself. His body had been under a tremendous amount of stress, and I felt I needed to be there to help him and hear each update from his transplant team.

Reid's parents drove back and forth to the hospital each day and spent the day there with us to help in any way possible. They didn't want to miss any moments of their son's recovery.

One morning, at 4 AM, a nurse walked in while Reid and I were still asleep and flipped all the lights on. In a loud voice, she announced, "I need to get your weight."

Reid snapped at her, "No, you don't. You can come back later. I'm not getting out of bed right now for that."

Reid had always been very cooperative and never snapped at others, so for him to do so showed me that he had to be in a good amount of pain, and the medications were still affecting his mental state. They had warned us the medication could have this effect, but Reid thought it wouldn't happen to him.

During that week, we received extensive post-transplant education. Tinker and I were required to attend a class to learn how to care for Reid after his transplant. At the class, we were given a three-ring binder full of information.

We reviewed each medication he was taking and which side effects and symptoms to look for. Upon release, he would be taking 21 oral pills each day. Every medication had its own side effects, so we needed to identify which side effects were alarming and when to call the transplant center. He would also need to swish his mouth after each meal with an antifungal, Nystatin.

We were given a vital signs log and instructed to check his blood pressure, temperature, and blood sugar multiple times daily. They told us he could no longer pick up dog poop, and Tinker swears she heard them say he couldn't change diapers when the babies were here. I certainly did not hear that part and still refuse to acknowledge it was ever said.

A pharmacist came by one day with an array of medication bottles and showed us which ones Reid would need each day. She told me I would need to refill and track his medication in the beginning until he got the hang of it, and then Reid could take over once we both felt comfortable. She instructed me to wear gloves any time I touched his medications, as some of them could pass through my skin and be harmful to the babies.

It was completely overwhelming and there was a lot of information to take in, but I felt well-organized and confident in our ability to handle the new routine.

On January 21st, one week after his transplant, they released Reid to go home. His liver numbers looked great. I now know that he had been in immense pain based on everything that unfolded in the next 24 hours. He did not express to anyone how much pain he was experiencing because he assumed the pain was a normal part of recovery after a liver transplant.

He hadn't had a bowel movement since the surgery, but he had been on a liquid diet for four of those days, so we assumed maybe that was normal. As solid foods were introduced to his system, pressure started to build in his abdomen. Reid didn't voice it, but he felt nervous about leaving the hospital. He knew I wasn't sleeping great in the hospital recliner, but he also knew I would not go home without him. I think he had become eager for me to get home and sleep in our own bed despite how much pain he was in.

That night at home, however, neither of us got any sleep. Reid had so much pain in his abdomen, and we didn't know what was going on. He felt as though his stomach was stretched as big as it could get, and each breath he took pulled on the 42 staples that held his incision together. *Was this normal transplant pain? Or was something wrong?*

The next morning, his stomach was so bloated and full that it felt like food was coming back up his throat. By 10 AM, he couldn't even drink water, and we feared he wouldn't keep his transplant medication down. He started hiccupping, which pulled on the staples across his incisions each time. It felt as though he were wearing a belt around his belly that radiated pain across his entire midsection every time he hiccupped or moved.

Reid's parents came over, and we all decided to call his transplant coordinator. They instructed us to come into the clinic to be evaluated by the transplant team.

When we arrived at the hospital clinic, and Reid's transplant coordinator saw how much pain he was in, she immediately called the transplant floor to see if they had a bed for him. They did not and wouldn't for a while, so she sent him straight to the ER for immediate attention.

Reid's dad pushed him in a wheelchair as we headed down to the ER, and I called Tinker. She had run home to grab an overnight bag while Ric and I drove Reid to the hospital. After the night we had, we knew I would need to come back home to sleep, and Reid would likely be admitted, so his mom offered to stay with him.

When we arrived at the check-in desk at the ER, I told the receptionist where we had come from and that Reid's transplant team said he needed to be seen immediately. I looked around and realized the waiting room was overflowing, and patients were lying on gurneys in the hallway because they were completely full.

By the time we finally got a "room" (if you can call it that) in the ER, Reid's mom had arrived at the hospital. The pain had become unbearable, and Reid pleaded for someone to help him.

As each minute passed, I became more concerned. I begged the hospital staff to do something to ease his pain, but they didn't have the resources to cover everyone.

Eight hours after arriving at the hospital, they finally performed a CT scan and were able to transfer Reid up to a room on the transplant floor. I headed home because I could feel the stress taking a toll on me. I wanted so badly to be there with my husband to support him, but I also needed to take care of our babies, and I desperately needed sleep. Ric drove me home while Tinker stayed behind with Reid.

Reid had been in pain and hiccupping non-stop for 12 hours by the time he arrived on the transplant floor. The team placed an NG tube in to attempt to alleviate some of the pressure Reid was feeling in his abdomen. Right after his transplant, the NG tube made him miserable, and he couldn't wait to get it out. This time, he begged them to put one in as he knew it would be so much better than the pain he was feeling. As the tube went in, he immediately started to feel some of the fluid being pulled out and some pressure being relieved, which allowed his body to relax a little.

They learned through the CT scan that he had an ileus, which meant a blockage was preventing movement through his intestines. But the CT couldn't tell them the cause of the ileus. They had to put him back into surgery to find the source and fix it.

Thankfully, his entire transplant team came in to do that surgery. They knew he was still in a critical time for his recovery and wanted to make sure this surgery didn't affect his new organ.

Tinker sat in the waiting room alone in the middle of the night as they wheeled him back to the OR. I was home doing my best to sleep while I knew my husband was undergoing surgery, waking up often to check my phone for updates.

The exact recounts of that night weren't shared with me for obvious reasons until later. But the terror Reid's mom felt, fearing her son wouldn't survive the night while I slept to protect our babies, is a mother's worst nightmare. She had already been through hell during the transplant, but that night put her through the wringer once again. It took an incredibly long time to find the source of the ileus, and as each minute ticked by, Tinker became more worried. *Four hours* after they had taken him back for surgery, one of the transplant surgeons came out to the waiting room.

Tinker had her face buried in her hands and tears streaming down her face. She was in a smaller waiting room, as the large one wasn't open in the middle of the night. It was dark and only had eight chairs, but she was the only one in the room. Dr. Moore walked over to her and asked her, "Are you okay?"

"No," she admitted, terrified of what the surgeon would say next.

Dr. Moore shared they had finally found the source of the ileus. Scar tissue from his appendectomy years prior had wrapped around the intestines, closing off movement through them. The doctor told her that the surgery was simple once they found the problem and that Reid should be okay. With this issue corrected, he could start to heal.

*Thank you, Jesus.*

We mentally prepared for another hospital stay, this time with Reid much more comfortable. He spent the first few days in the ICU, and I traveled back and forth to our house each night to sleep. I stopped by to get the mail one evening, and there was a large manilla envelope addressed to Reid. I opened it to find cards from the first-grade class that my friend Hollie taught. I brought the cards to Reid the next morning, and he read each of them, amazed at the kindness of these children who didn't even know him.

After another week-long stay in the hospital, Reid was back home to recover. Our amazing support system came through for us again. They brought prepared food and groceries, sent care packages, came over and helped with things around the house, and checked in on us regularly. Reid's recovery progressed daily, and seeing how much better he felt was incredible.

On February 20th, I had an appointment with my doctor, who specialized in high-risk pregnancies. She checked on the babies and did all the measurements. When she measured my cervix, it had shortened to a point where she was concerned about early labor. She rechecked it just to be sure and immediately said she wanted me admitted to the hospital.

She called my regular OB-GYN and discussed her concerns. They agreed I could be admitted to the hospital near our home, and he would oversee my care for this stay. They both knew Reid was at home recovering from a liver transplant and still not able to drive. They understood that being at a hospital closer to home was the best option.

They weren't overly concerned about me going into labor right then, but they were concerned enough to have me monitored and start a magnesium drip to slow down contractions (which I didn't even realize I was having). The doctor also ordered steroid shots to help the babies' lungs develop should they come early.

At this point, Reid's recovery had been going well. His liver numbers looked great, and he had weekly appointments with his transplant team. But we desperately needed the babies to stay put a little longer.

After a few days in the hospital, they released me to go home on bed rest. My high-risk doctor said we would follow up later that week, but I had strict orders to stay on bed rest for the remainder of the pregnancy.

So there we were: five weeks post-transplant, 26 weeks pregnant, and I was being put on bed rest. If there had ever been a time we needed to depend on everyone around us, this was it. We were quite the helpless pair – neither of us could even take out the trash – but all our dreams were coming true, and we were so close to holding our babies in our arms.

And Reid would be here for that moment.

# Chapter 28

## We Meet Larry and Beth Sparks

### Spring 2019

We caught up on a lot of TV during this time. Reid got up and moved around more, which the doctors encouraged, so he could at least cook for us and help with some light things around the house. He had just returned to work part-time when I was put on bedrest, so he switched to working remotely to be at home with me during the day.

We went from me taking care of him to him taking care of me. Our support team sat on high alert, checking on the two of us daily. I honestly don't know how we would have gotten through those days without his parents, who seemed to be at our house almost every day helping with something.

Every week or two, one of my doctors admitted me to the hospital with pre-labor scares, and then I would be sent home a few days later. Despite that, as each week passed, we celebrated that our babies had stayed put for a little longer.

We had talked to Beth and Larry Sparks a few times, and I gave Beth updates via text on how Reid and I were doing.

About a week after Reid's transplant, he and I decided we wanted to use Clayton as a middle name for our son. We had always been set on our daughter's name – Kaylee June (June was my Mema's middle name), and we knew we wanted our son's name to be Oliver, but we couldn't agree on a middle name. Now we knew why. Fate already knew his name: Oliver Clayton.

One night, I texted Beth and asked if she and Larry could talk. The four of us got on a phone call, and Reid and I told them we wanted to name our son Oliver Clayton. We heard silence on the phone for a moment, and then, "Yes, we would love that," through sobs. Clayton saved my husband, and we wanted our kids to always know his name and what he did for us. Using Clayton as a middle name was our way of honoring their son and his incredible gift to our family.

On April 6th, we finally met Beth and Larry in person. They drove the 40 minutes to our house with Clayton's uncle, best friend, and girlfriend. We also had Ric and Tinker, my mom, and my stepdad at our house to meet them.

I had difficulty sitting still in the hours leading up to that meeting. I wanted so badly to get up and clean just to keep my mind busy, but I knew I needed to stick to my bedrest limitations as much as possible. Our parents came over that morning and ensured the house was clean and ready for guests. I tried my best to relax, but my nervous system was in overdrive.

We couldn't wait to meet these amazing people, but I also needed this important and delicate meeting to go well. They were coming to our house to meet us because their son died. And in his death, he saved my husband.

How do you even find the words to express gratitude for such a gift? Would one of us say the wrong thing? What frame of mind would Beth and Larry be in? Would they resent my husband for being alive while their son was not? Is it okay to be happy and celebrate this gift, or is that disrespectful as they still grieve their son?

All I knew about this kind of meeting was what I had seen on social media…you know, those videos that bring tears to your eyes when a donor family meets the organ recipient. Should I video this? Is that awkward? How would they feel about that? I asked my stepdad to video as they arrived at our house, but to also be sure to read the room and turn the video off if it felt awkward. We've never shared that video, but it is now a precious memory.

From the first time meeting the Sparks, I knew they would be a big part of our family. We all had many things in common, and our meeting only brought more similarities to our attention. We brought a few kitchen chairs to the living room and made a circle, including our sectional couch. The room was filled with both joy and sadness as we listened to so many stories about Clayton and the amazing things he did during his time here on Earth. We learned how Clayton constantly thought of others and inspired his friends to do the same.

From a young age, he worried about other kids who may not get much at Christmas. He stayed up late one night and wrote letters to his friends, which he delivered at school the next day, requesting his friends bring gifts for those less fortunate. He then dressed up as Santa Claus and delivered gifts to the needy.

Each year, he asked for money instead of gifts for his birthday. He then went grocery shopping and delivered all the items he purchased with his birthday money to the local food bank.

Clayton loved wearing Hawaiian shirts, so all of his friends wore Hawaiian shirts to his funeral.

He was the life of the party and a friend to everyone he met.

The more we talked and learned about him, the more we understood how great this loss was for Clayton's family and friends. And the more our families felt intertwined.

Tears brought us together, but we found laughter and joy through those tears.

# Chapter 29

## More Miracles – Oliver Clayton and Kaylee June

### April 2019

On April 11th, five days after meeting the Sparks family, my mom arrived at our house to take me to an appointment with my high-risk doctor. As she walked in, she called out, "Abby? You here?"

"In here," I responded from my bedroom. I sat on the edge of our bedframe with an unsure look on my face. "I'm either peeing myself, or my water just broke," I told her.

Her face lit up as we both started laughing. "Oh my gosh! Really?" the excitement in her voice was palpable.

Reid heard the commotion from the living room and walked in to see what was happening as I shuffled back into the bathroom. I yelled to my mom and Reid, "Yeah, it's not stopping! My water definitely broke!"

I grabbed the thickest pad I could find, which was quickly replaced by a baby diaper that my mom grabbed from our stash, and changed out of my soaking wet pants. I called my doctor's office, and they told me to head straight to the hospital. Dr. Aron, my high-risk doctor, would meet me there. I wasn't having contractions, at least none that I felt, but these babies were ready to get things moving.

We quickly jumped in the car (with many towels in my seat) and headed to the medical center. I was 33 weeks, five days along in the pregnancy.

Our little miracle babies wanted to meet us six weeks early.

I knew this meant they would require a stay in the NICU, but I also knew the babies were at a point where they weren't considered so premature that it was a huge worry.

I called a few of our family and friends to let them know my water broke. I asked them to sit tight because we weren't sure when the babies would arrive.

No one listened.

Soon, we had a full hospital room: my mom, my dad, my mother-in-law and father-in-law, my sister, my best friend, and my aunt. And then my grandma walked in pushing her husband in a wheelchair… she had driven an hour and a half to be there.

We had all anxiously awaited this moment for so long, and none of them were going to miss the day that our dream of becoming parents finally became a reality.

Several long hours passed as we waited for Dr. Aron to visit and decide whether to proceed with delivery. When she finally came by, she stared at the toco reading, which recorded my contractions, and debated. "I'm not sure we're ready to deliver," she told me.

"Are you serious? These babies are ready. I'm ready." I argued.

She reluctantly agreed to perform the c-section that night. As they wheeled me into the OR, I looked at the clock, which showed almost midnight; it was just a few hours away from the anniversary of Reid and I meeting for our blind date. I debated asking her to hold off until midnight so they could arrive exactly eight years from the day we met, but I decided not to since I had already pushed to have the c-section that night.

As they finished my spinal block, the doctor walked into the OR. "Please make sure they're born on the same day. If you can't deliver them both before midnight, then let's hold off so they don't have two different birthdays," I pleaded.

"Why do you think I'm rushing? Everyone ready? Let's go." She ordered.

At 11:48 and 11:49 PM, Oliver Clayton and Kaylee June arrived via c-section. As they took Oliver from my uterus, Dr. Aron said, "Baby A is out; now let's get Baby B."

"Wait, he's out? He's not crying! Why isn't he crying??" I begged as tears streamed down my face. I looked up at Reid with pleading eyes. *Tell me our baby is okay.*

Just then, we heard the most beautiful sound. The one we'd been waiting so many years to hear. Our baby crying. The NICU team grabbed him since he was having a little trouble breathing, but they assured me he was okay; he just needed a little oxygen.

Before I could fully register our baby boy was here, we heard a second baby crying. This one had a tiny voice with a little shriek to it. Our baby girl. She came out fiery and ready to make her presence known.

I looked up at Reid and said, "Can you see them? Are they okay?"

I could see his smile around the surgical mask as he said, "They're okay."

The nurse who had performed my spinal tap leaned over my head and said, "They're cleaning up both babies, and then you can see them. You did great."

I sobbed, so eager to see their sweet faces and hold them, but my hands were strapped to the arms of the table as they finished closing my abdomen.

They brought Kaylee over for Reid to hold. He put her next to my head as I lay on the operating table. I studied her sweet face and cried. After a minute, they took her away and brought Oliver over to repeat the same process. I looked at his face in awe. My breath quickened as I tried to hold back more tears.

Our precious babies were here.

Both babies were healthy but needed to stay in the NICU to "feed and grow."

The first couple of days in the hospital after their birth were a whirlwind as I functioned on auto-pilot, trying to recover and see the babies as much as possible. Reid wheeled me down to the NICU often to see them, and I pumped breast milk every two hours to get my supply built up.

The first time I held them, it felt like a dream. This had to be someone else's life, not mine. I looked down at each of them, tears rolling down my face.

Kaylee weighed a delicate 4 pounds 6 ounces. She had petite features and big, beautiful eyes. Like Reid and me, she had long fingers and toes.

Oliver weighed 6 pounds 8 ounces and had a grumpy demeanor. He had been hogging most of the nutrients from his sister, and she had obviously been kicking him in the face while they were in utero, as he came out with bruises.

From the first day of meeting them, I felt they each had a unique personality, and I loved that about them.

All of our parents came by to see the babies on the first day, and I will never forget the feeling of watching Tinker, Ric, my mom, and my dad meet their grandbabies for the first time. Seeing their love for our babies filled my heart so much that it could have burst out of my chest.

They had been alongside us for the entire fight. They saw us at our worst and cried with us during each of the losses. Our amazing parents prayed and fought and grieved for the last four years as we tried so hard to become a family.

Holding the babies wasn't an easy task because of all the wires and monitors they were hooked up to, but I was determined to let our parents hold them.

Growing up, I was close with all my grandparents, and I know first-hand what a special bond that is. I couldn't wait to see all of them develop that bond with our babies.

Dr. Aron released me from the hospital a few days later. I was glad to go home and sleep in our own bed, but I hated the thought of leaving the hospital without our precious babies.

Reid came with me to the hospital for the first few days, but then he had to return to work. He had missed so much work already that year, and we wanted to save his time off for when Kaylee and Oliver got to come home.

My team had not cleared me to drive yet, so my father-in-law, Ric, drove me to the medical center daily and spent the entire day there with the babies and me. He helped feed and change them and took my breast milk to the milk bank after I pumped. Tinker came to help on the days she wasn't working, and on the weekends, my mom and sister came to help and see the babies.

I thought at that point we had been through the hardest part of our journey – and we had. But it didn't make it any easier having to leave my babies in the care of others as I went home each night to sleep.

I was still recovering from my c-section, but I put a lot of pressure on myself to be at the hospital as much as possible. We would leave the house by 7 AM each morning and come home around 7 PM every night.

I cried every day as we left the hospital, and my sweet father-in-law would talk me through it the whole way home. Leaving the hospital each day meant leaving a piece of myself behind.

I wanted my babies to be home with us so badly, but they weren't ready. Each night, I called the NICU nurse around 2 AM to check on Kaylee and Oliver as I sat in our living room connected to a breast pump.

Every day felt like a roller coaster as they tracked each feeding for the babies, and it often felt like we were taking one step forward and two steps back.

Kaylee was having "bradys," where her heart rate would dip, and the monitor would go crazy, sending us all into a panic. We couldn't take her home while this was still happening.

The NICU team discussed Oliver coming home, but Kaylee wasn't ready. That completely broke my heart. How could I take one of our twins home and leave the other at a hospital 40 minutes away?

Reid took a day off work for his weekly appointment with the transplant team, so he came to spend the day in the NICU with me and the babies. When it was time for his appointment, he walked down the street to the hospital transplant center. He came back a little later and offered to feed the babies while I went and grabbed some lunch.

As he was feeding Kaylee, his transplant coordinator called and told him, "Grab a mask. Don't touch any surfaces, and head directly back to the hospital admissions desk at Methodist."

His bloodwork had come back, and his immune system had tanked. His levels were dangerously low. They feared he would easily pick up any germs, which would attack his system without any defense. They needed to admit him into the hospital to do some treatments and keep him safe.

I returned to the NICU just as he finished his phone call, and he explained what the nurse had just told him.

This sent me into a spiral. My chest tightened, and my palms started to sweat. I tried to hold my tears back as Reid quickly hugged me, grabbed a mask, and left.

There I sat with two newborn babies in the NICU, and now they were admitting my husband into the hospital because his immune system had overreacted to his immuno-suppressants. I broke down as soon as Reid left, and the floodgates burst open.

Our amazing NICU nurse, Patricia, came over and sat beside me as I cried. She hugged me and assured me everyone would be okay. She talked me through the situation and helped me see the logical side. Patricia went above and beyond her job description, and I am forever thankful for her.

The three people I loved most in this world were in the hospital, but her talk reminded me that I had the strength to get through this, just as I had with everything else we'd been through.

The NICU doctor came by a little later and told me Oliver could go home in the next day or two. While I felt grateful for that news, I didn't know how I was going to juggle having one baby at home, one in the hospital, and my husband in a different hospital.

Patricia explained our situation to the doctor, and they agreed it would be best to keep Oliver in the NICU for a few more days. Hopefully, Kaylee would be ready to come home by then. *Please, God. Let Reid come home soon, too.* I wanted my babies home together, but I also wanted their dad to be there.

The next day, my mom went with me to the NICU to visit the babies. As soon as I arrived, I told the nurses I wanted to do skin-to-skin with both babies. Skin-to-skin is when the baby is wearing a diaper without any other clothes, and you remove your shirt so there is direct skin contact as you hold the baby. Doing this with newborns has many benefits, one being that it calms the mother and baby.

With two babies in the NICU, skin-to-skin was not an easy task. They both had monitors attached to them, and their cribs were across from each other, so my chair had to be positioned right in between to allow their cords to reach back to the machines to which they were attached. It took me, my mom, and two nurses to get us situated, but we did it.

They laid both babies on my bare chest and then wrapped a blanket around the three of us.

Once we were situated, my entire body relaxed, and my emotions took over. Tears started rolling down my face. At that moment, reality hit me. Everything we prayed for had come true, but in a way we never expected.

For so many years, we fought hard. We fought for Reid's health. We fought to have babies. And now we had it all.

Yes, Reid was in the hospital, still fighting to be healthy, but he would be okay. And our babies were here and in my arms. Sitting there holding my miracle babies felt like an out-of-body experience.

My mom saw the tears streaming down my face and came over to check on me. She stroked my hair as my tears turned to sobs, and I whispered, "This is it. I can't believe we made it." She started crying with me, and we both just soaked in the emotions of that moment.

The following day, after receiving two days of Granix injections to boost his body's production of white blood cells, Reid came home from the hospital. The day after that, our babies were discharged. Ric went with me to pick up Kaylee and Oliver so Reid could stay home and recover from his hospital stay.

I remember riding in the back of the car with the babies, wondering if this is what all new parents feel when bringing their babies home—a mix of joy and terror.

Our babies were coming home, and my husband was a transplant recipient and getting healthier every day.

Miracles do exist—we are living proof of that.

# Chapter 30

## Our New Normal

### 2019-2021

The first year of the twins' lives felt like it had gone by in a blur.

I remember sitting on the couch and crying while I held them because I felt so grateful they were here. But then there were times I would sit and cry from complete exhaustion as I wondered how I could continue to juggle taking care of two babies at once.

We had survived an incredibly tough journey and made it through. Certainly, we could make it through the hard newborn days as well. We were okay. But were we? Was *I* really okay?

I often found myself filled with intense anxiety, fearing something terrible would happen. After all we had been through, how could we get everything we'd dreamed of for so long? Surely, the next bomb would be dropping soon.

When my sister and I were both pregnant, I was in disbelief that everything would work out as we hoped. I couldn't wrap my head around the fact that we were both having boy/girl twins three months apart. During our pregnancies, I feared something would happen to one of our four babies, and we would be experiencing immeasurable grief.

For so long, all I had known was pain and heartbreak, but three months after we had Oliver and Kaylee, Maddox and Mallie were born.

I gave birth to our twins at 33 weeks, five days… Megan gave birth to hers at 33 weeks, six days. I joked with my sister it wasn't enough for her to get pregnant with twins her first month of trying; she had to keep them in a day longer, too.

But seriously, the only thing that mattered was they were here and healthy. Her twins also had a NICU stay, and we helped my sister and her husband through that as much as we could.

Everyone loves a good newborn snuggle, so it was no surprise many of our friends and family wanted to come over to meet our tiny miracle babies. They had all been praying for our family for so long that I felt obligated to invite these wonderful people, who supported us unconditionally, to meet the twins.

But before anyone arrived at our home, my anxiety would take over. As soon as they walked in the door, I instructed them to take their shoes off and wash their hands before properly greeting them. Then, for their entire visit, I would take note of which surfaces they touched so I could clean those spots as soon as they left. There were a few times I even changed the babies' clothes after having visitors.

My husband had an immuno-compromised body due to his anti-rejection medications, so I worried he would pick up an illness that would compromise his new liver. I also acted as the "germ police" because the babies had been in the NICU for 19 days, where they instructed us to wash our hands often and sanitize before and after each activity.

I used to love having visitors in our home, but after everything we'd been through, it would now send me into an internal spiral.

However, our amazing support team had been a part of our journey to get here, and I wanted them to see our precious miracles, so I had to try my best to put aside my fears. Our babies were surrounded by so much love, even before they were born, and I wanted them to feel that.

When Oliver and Kaylee were around seven months old, Reid had surgery to repair an abdominal hernia, which was left over from the transplant. He couldn't lift the babies (or anything over five pounds) for three months. Having that restriction proved to be quite hard on both of us.

Then, when the twins received their one-year immunizations, Reid had to leave the house for two weeks as the kids had received live vaccinations. Since the vaccines were live, his transplant team feared he could be exposed to the weakened strains of the diseases the vaccines were meant to fight, which is unsafe for those with compromised immune systems.

These are the things that come with transplant life. The entire family is affected, and we must always make adjustments to ensure Reid is okay. Issues with his health will inevitably come up from time to time. But those sacrifices are minor in comparison to the alternative.

In January of 2020, I wrote and shared the following blog post:

*Over the last few months, I've dealt with some severe anxiety. And I've avoided sharing. Because I had babies recently, there is often the response of, "You're a new mom. It's normal to have anxiety." And that's true. It is expected to have "new mom" anxiety and to have a new level of stress that comes with raising tiny humans. However, what I've been dealing with is so much more.*

*I wake up in the middle of the night with a pit in my stomach and have to catch my breath. I often think about losing my husband or one of our babies, and I spiral into a puddle of anxiety. Every time I walk up and down the stairs with a baby in my arms, I am anxious they will suddenly throw themselves out of my arms and go over the railing. If Reid doesn't do something for the babies the exact way I would have done, I become angry. Any time someone walks into my house, I have severe anxiety watching any surface they touch before they wash their hands so I can be sure to clean it later. Every time I get in the car, I think about how terrible it would be if I were to get in a wreck. I could go on and on with the millions of scenarios that have gone through my head. It's not normal. It's consuming. It's exhausting. And it's been affecting my entire family.*

*Over the holidays, it got particularly bad. As we prepared to see more friends and family, I got more anxious, knowing someone could pass on an illness to my husband or babies. As I thought about those experiencing their first holiday season without their loved ones, I became anxious because I felt I could never survive that. Then, I became anxious again that I was going to miss out on opportunities to make Oliver & Kaylee's first Christmas as special as possible because I was so ridden with anxiety. Do you see the spiral? As I type it, it feels crazy. I feel crazy. One day, I couldn't get out of bed and finally told Reid, "I can't kick this on my own. I need professional help."*

*I saw a psychiatrist on January 15th. And there, I laid out our story.*

*It will probably come as no surprise I have been diagnosed with PTSD (Post Traumatic Stress Disorder) and anxiety, and my psychiatrist also believes that I have developed some OCD (Obsessive-Compulsive Disorder) tendencies. I have started a few medications that are slowly starting to help, and I have been seeing a therapist weekly for talk therapy. I will also be doing EMDR (Eye Movement Desensitization and Reprocessing) therapy, which I hope will help.*

*It is a process. I wish so badly there was a quick fix, but I know first-hand that the things in life that are worth fighting for are usually not quick fixes. But we have worked so hard for everything we have now… I don't want to waste another second being anxious, sad, and angry. I want to be able to soak up every single second I have with the miracles we have received. I want to positively influence our children, my husband, our friends and family, and strangers who come across our story. And to do that, I have to love myself. I have to put the work in to make myself a better person. I need to give myself the grace that I deserve to work through the very tough things we've overcome over the last few years. I have to admit that it's okay to not be okay. And I have to set an example for my kids that they would be proud of. Because mental health is so important, and it's not something to be ashamed of. I am struggling with PTSD and anxiety, but I am committed to doing the work to get through it. It will not consume me and take over my life, as hard as it may try.*

I felt like a terrible person, so ridden with guilt. We had received everything we had fought for, and I wasn't fully enjoying it.

Family and friends would tell me to soak up the little moments, and they would say, "The days are long, but the years are short." Those words only reminded me that I was letting this time slip away.

We had been through so much and made it to the other side. I understood the breakdowns along our journey, but why was I breaking down *now*?

In hindsight, it all makes sense to me. My sole focus had been getting through the challenges we had in front of us. For four years, we had fought for our family. I worked to keep it all together the best I could so we could continue fighting, but a person can only operate that way for so long.

Sustaining a life of constantly battling trauma is bound to catch up with anyone, and that's exactly what it did for me. Even though, at times, I felt I was dealing with my emotions and processing them with different therapists, a part of me had been avoiding truly seeing how complex the challenges in front of us were.

Reid's biggest concern was always *me*. He knew I had been spiraling downward into a bad place and wanted to support me however he could.

Shortly after I started seeing both a psychiatrist and a therapist regularly, the COVID pandemic of 2020 hit. So many people struggled during that time with isolation from family and friends or even being able to make a regular run to the grocery store.

For me, though, quarantine was exactly what I needed. It allowed me to stay put in my safe bubble without judgment while I processed all that had happened during the previous few years. It provided the opportunity to focus solely on the three people I had fought so hard for. The seclusion allowed me to heal.

I am not in any way saying the COVID pandemic was a good thing; I know people who lost loved ones to COVID-19, and being quarantined was incredibly hard for so many. But being secluded with my immediate family gave me peace and time to rest and mend internally.

A silver lining from this period is that it offered a glimpse into the life of transplant patients and the precautions they must take daily to keep themselves healthy. Everyone, not only transplant patients, had to be careful during this time.

Reid worked from home during the pandemic, and having him there in our safe bubble was so nice.

I have so many videos on my phone of our family of four laughing and playing together during our quarantine. I slowly let my guard down and began to find joy again in the little moments, shifting my focus away from all the potential things that could go wrong.

Our neighbors had an immuno-compromised son and were taking extra precautions, so we developed a strong bond with their family. Their grandson is only two months older than Oliver and Kaylee, so we were able to have some playtime for the kids without the extra risk of the outside world. I grew close with their daughter and found an incredible new friend in her.

I called at least one set of grandparents each day, and we would sit on video chat while Oliver and Kaylee played. We were able to actually have some good conversations that didn't focus on medical issues and stress.

The twins had their first birthday during our quarantine. While it made me sad we couldn't be with our family and friends to celebrate this huge milestone, we celebrated through Zoom and made the best of it.

We were living the life we dreamed of for so long. Yet, I still carried underlying anxiety that, at any moment, Reid would be taken down with an illness, and his compromised body wouldn't recover. I feared something would happen to one or both of our twins, and we'd experience great loss.

I was regularly overcome with fear that one of my loved one's hearts would suddenly stop, and I often woke in the middle of the night to lay a hand on Reid's chest and make sure his heart was still beating. Then, I would stare at the baby monitor as I watched our babies' chests rise and fall before I could fall back asleep.

I continued working closely with my therapist to develop more coping skills to adjust to our new normal. We adjusted the EMDR sessions so that they could be done virtually, and I'm so glad that was an option because EMDR made a huge difference for me.

In the fall of 2021, we enrolled Oliver and Kaylee in a nearby "Mother's Day Out" program two days a week. They were two years old, and I knew school would be good for them, but putting them in a more public environment also made me nervous.

Everyone assured me it would be the best thing for all of us, and they were right. As a stay-at-home mom, the days the twins were in school allowed me to get some things done around our house and have some "me" time.

Reid will always be immuno-compromised, and our family must always be more diligent about germs and contact with others. But I knew we couldn't live in our bubble forever. Our kids bring us so much happiness; I want to share that joy with others. That meant finding a balance. We continue to work hard to be careful about what we can control while living our lives.

These days, we don't miss those important events, but you will always find me pushing Reid to the front of the line at family gatherings so he can get his food before everyone else has their hands in it. I am diligent about reminding him to wash his hands. Our children know they need to take extra caution with germs as well, and this will be something they grow to understand more as they get older.

Reid has had some minor bumps along the way, but he is active and healthy overall. Clayton's liver turned out to be the perfect match for him.

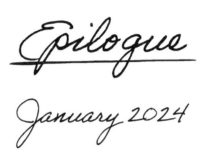

# Epilogue

## January 2024

"I give thanks for where my path has brought me" – that's what the sticky note on my desk reads.

I am so thankful for where we are today, but that doesn't negate our challenging journey to get here. I am committed to showing our gratitude without minimizing the struggle.

We recently celebrated Reid's fifth transplant anniversary. It's hard to comprehend how long it's been since that day.

I am sitting in my office as I write this, knowing that in the next 30 minutes, Oliver and Kaylee will greet me with a "Good morning, Mommy." Reid is working from home this morning, and they're always excited when they get to see Daddy in the mornings before school. This is their last year of preschool; they will turn five in a few months.

We won the jackpot with Oliver and Kaylee. They are two completely different individuals, and I love how well they complement each other.

Oliver is a jokester but also very analytical, just like his dad. He is an intelligent little boy who knew how to spell his name when he was two and can now rattle off square roots at almost five. He loves to make his sister (and anyone else who is around) laugh, and he will do something over and over *and over* again if she's laughing at him. He loves playing games and making puzzles and has inherited his dad's competitive nature. He is a helper and loves having a job.

Kaylee is kind and empathetic. She is artistic and always singing and dancing, without a care in the world for who may be watching or whether anyone else is joining her. Her kind and caring heart often has her worried about others. If her brother is upset, Kaylee will rush to his side to try and make him feel better. Her laugh is infectious, and it's obvious she's happy when she bounces around. She loves big and truly soaks in the little moments, which reminds us to do the same.

There are times Reid and I are in complete awe as we sit and watch them play. The children we prayed so hard for are here, healthy, and complete miracles.

Sometimes, I hear Reid playing with them in the next room, and the laughter stops me in my tracks. There were so many days when I wondered whether he would be here for moments like that, and hearing how much joy he brings them makes my heart swell.

We talk about Clayton often and refer to him as our family's superhero. One day, Kaylee told me that Clayton was our superhero because "Daddy fell into the lava, and Clayton came and saved him." I choked back tears as I stood there looking at my little miracle baby - who we were told was "incompatible with life" - craft this amazing story about how Clayton became our superhero.

Our relationship with Clayton's parents has grown into such a beautiful story of its own. Beth and Larry Sparks entered our lives through the transplant, but they have become an integral part of our family because they are wonderful people.

They are Oliver and Kaylee's additional set of grandparents, and they now go by BeBe and Pops to everyone in our extended family as well. The Sparks spend a lot of holidays with our family, and everyone loves having them around.

Oliver recently lost his first tooth, and when I asked if he wanted to call anyone to share the news, he asked to call BeBe and Pops. The kids enjoy frequent visits and love spending the night with them, often leading to them staying at their house for several days.

One day, a few months ago, the kids were at Beth and Larry's, and I called to do a video chat and say hi. While we were on the phone, Kaylee found a flower with a butterfly on it. She picked up the flower, but the butterfly didn't move, which was odd. Kaylee carried the flower over to show Oliver, and then the butterfly slowly moved from the flower to her arm. She continued to play as it sat on her arm the entire time. She's quite an active four-year-old, but the butterfly stayed with her. Kaylee was inside playing about 30 minutes later, and she told BeBe, "I think it's time for the butterfly to go back home now." She walked out the front door, and the butterfly flew away. Beth and I were both crying as we felt Clayton saying, "Thank you for being here."

We have had so many conversations with Beth and Larry, and they have shared how much their son being an organ donor has helped them in their grieving process. Clayton was incredibly kind and giving; this was his last gift to others. He continued to spread his kindness even after death, which gave them so much peace. By being an organ donor, Clayton significantly impacted the lives of 80 others.

I will never forget a conversation I had with Beth where I shared the guilt I felt about my husband still being alive while they no longer had their son. What she shared with me blew my mind. She said, "Abby, Clayton's accident would have happened whether Reid needed his liver or not. But the fact that we can see Clayton live on through Reid gives me joy I didn't even know was possible through losing my son."

The fact that Reid has made it to five years post-transplant is a pretty big deal. I mentioned earlier in the book that his disease – primary sclerosing cholangitis (PSC) – has a 40-60% chance of reoccurring in a new liver. New studies have shown that the chance of reoccurrence *significantly* drops at the five-year mark after transplant.

Over the last several years, in the back of my mind, I worried that he would be diagnosed with PSC again and we'd start the whole process over. I'm so grateful he has reached this pivotal milestone.

I have yet to go back to working full-time. I never thought I'd be a stay-at-home mom. I enjoyed having a job and growing my career, but I think our struggles changed my perspective. I want to soak up every (sometimes challenging, but mostly good) moment with my kids. They currently attend preschool four days a week, so I get to do drop-offs and pick-ups, and then we spend Fridays together.

Most days, I am still in disbelief that our story turned out the way it did. If someone had told me that shortly after we were married, we would experience the most difficult challenges (more than some go through in a lifetime) but also have the most incredible conclusion, I wouldn't have believed them.

I truly believe we have lived our story in order to share it with others, and I have made it my mission to do so. There were so many days when I was sure we would *never* get positive news. But in 2019, our world completely changed.

We were fortunate to have the support that we did throughout this process because I know many people don't. Reflecting on our journey, I know how incredibly blessed we were to receive such miracles. I also recognize how privileged we were to have so many resources available to us. I now aim to help as many people as possible experiencing similar struggles.

Reid and I are grateful you took the time to read our story. I hope you take away the following: Miracles do exist, hope is never lost, and good people around you want to help.

Expect miracles. A grateful heart is a magnet for miracles.

# Photos of our Journey

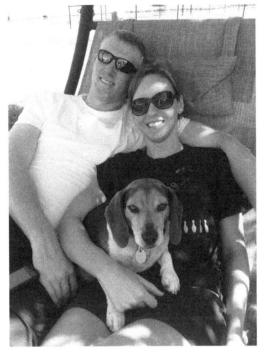

*Our first trip to Indiana to meet Reid's parents.*

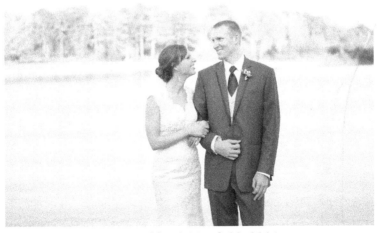

*Our wedding! March 29, 2014*

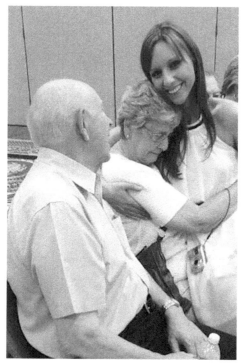

*Me and my Mema during rehearsal dinner. She was always
the first to cry tears of joy, and I loved that about her.*

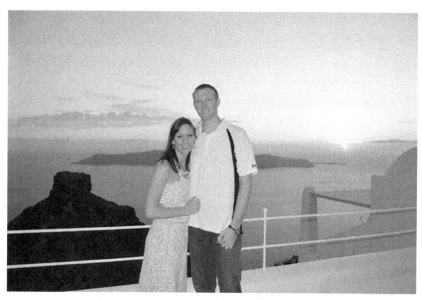

*On our honeymoon in beautiful Santorini.*

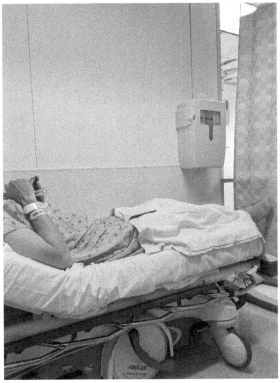

*Waiting for one of Reid's many procedures to check the status of his PSC & UC.*

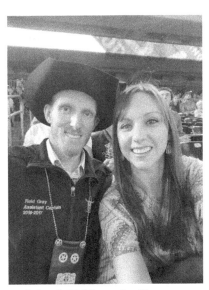

*March 2018, at the Houston Livestock Show and Rodeo after Reid's first hospitalization.*

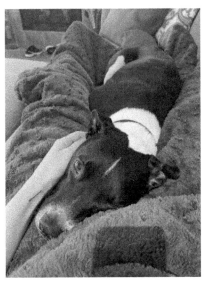

*Our sweet Wrigley giving me couch cuddles. He was the best cuddler.*

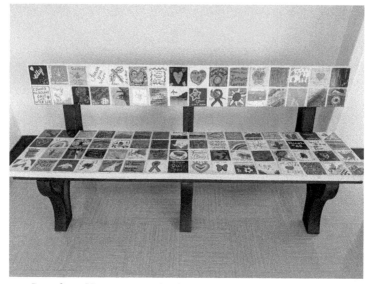

*Bench at Houston Methodist J.C. Walter Jr. Transplant Center honors loved ones who became organ donors.*

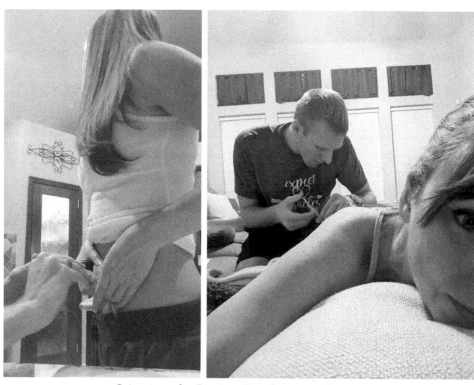

*Injections for In-vitro Fertilization (IVF).*

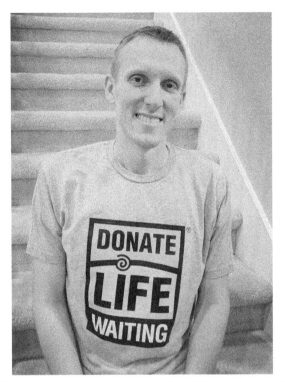

*Waiting for a liver transplant, and continuing to get sicker.*

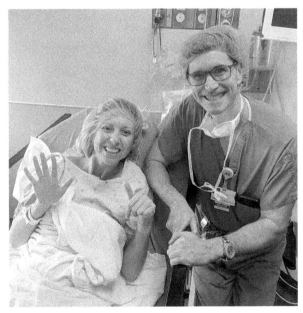

*Our third embryo retrieval, with the amazing Dr. Griffith.*

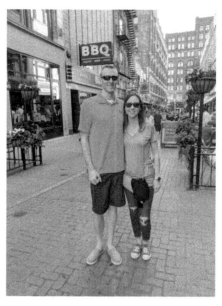

*Enjoying our time in Cleveland, in
between hospital appointments.*

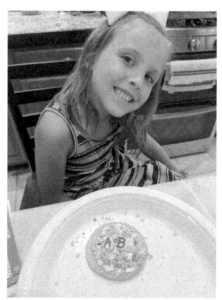

*Monroe, my best friend's daughter, with the "AB" cookies she made for me
and baby. Little did she know they really meant "Baby A" and "Baby B".*

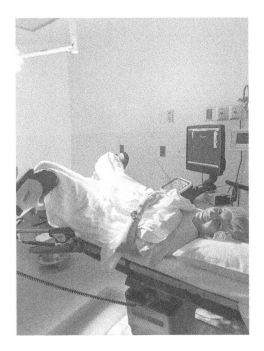

*Transferring our final two embryos.*

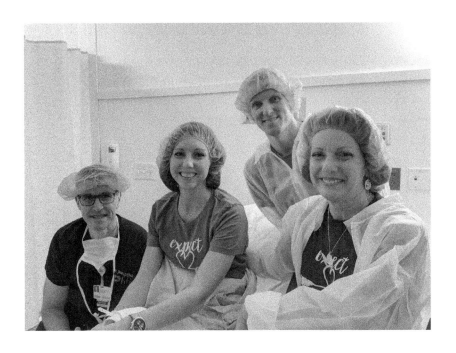

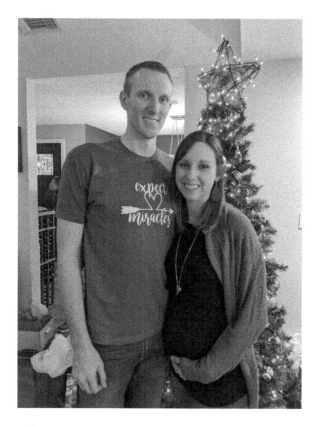

*Christmas 2018 with family. Everyone wore their*
*Expect Miracles shirts to show their support.*

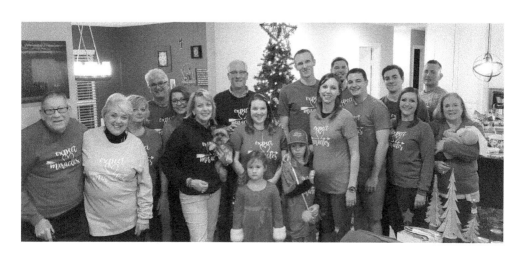

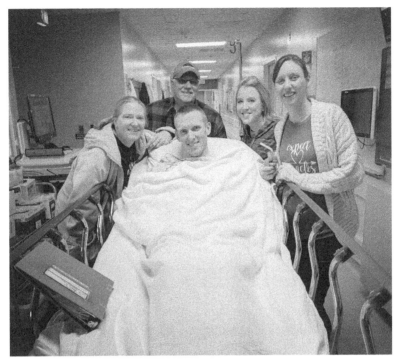

*The last picture we took right before they took Reid back to surgery.*

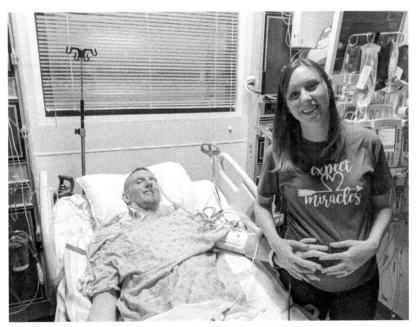

*A few days after Reid's transplant.*

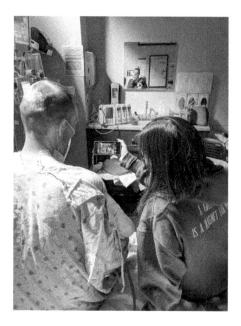

*Watching the video Clayton's friends and family sent us and looking at all of the cards that Hollie's class made for Reid.*

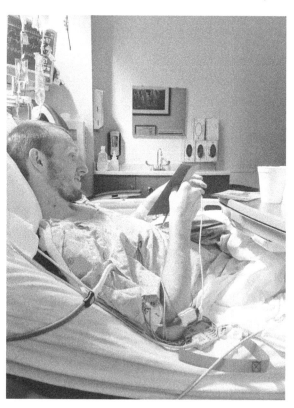

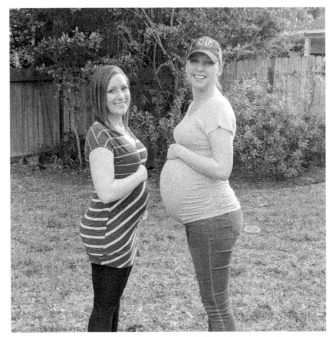

*My sister and I pregnant with twins together.*

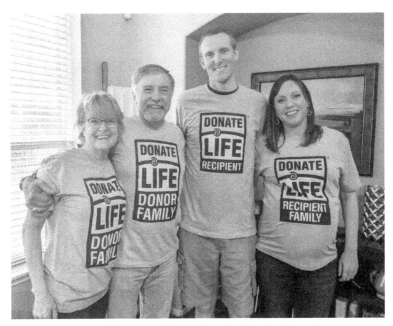

*We meet Larry and Beth Sparks for the first time.*

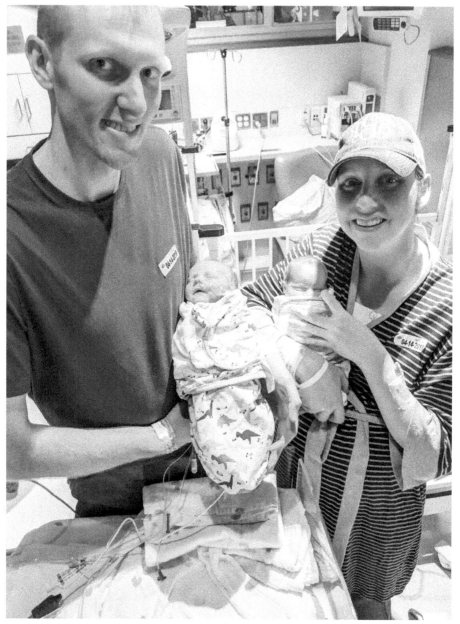

*The twins are born. This is our first photo as a family of four.*

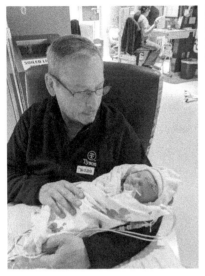
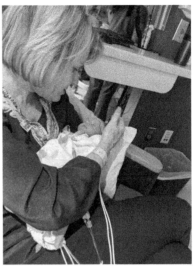

*Grandparents holding the babies for the first time.*

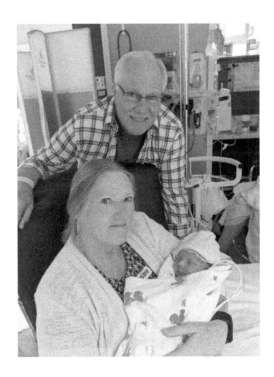

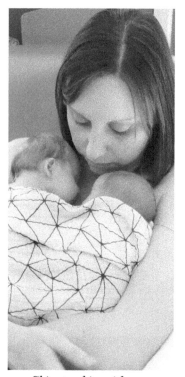

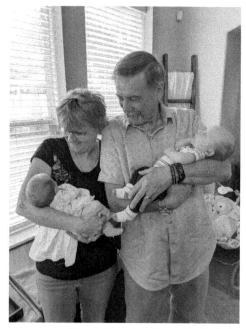

*Skin-to-skin with our miracle babies.*

*Larry and Beth Sparks (Pops & BeBe) meeting the twins for the first time.*

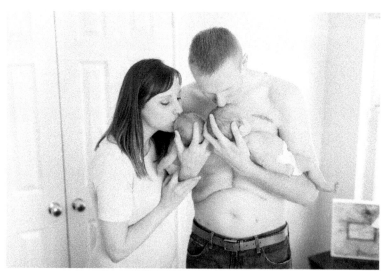

*Our first professional family photos with Sarah Ainsworth Photography. This perfectly captures our miracles in one photo.*

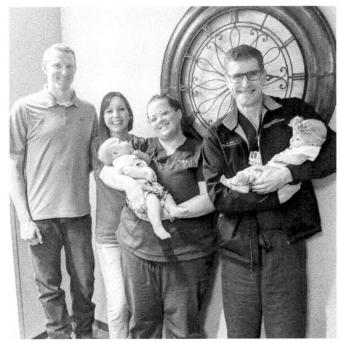

*Oliver & Kaylee are introduced to the team that never gave up on them.*

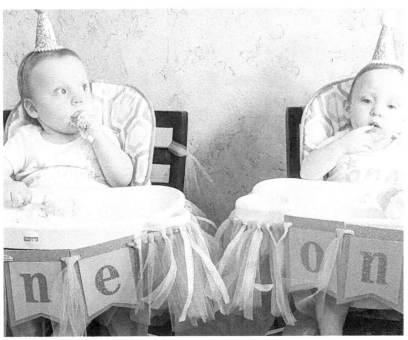

*The twins first birthday, celebrated via Zoom with our family and friends.*

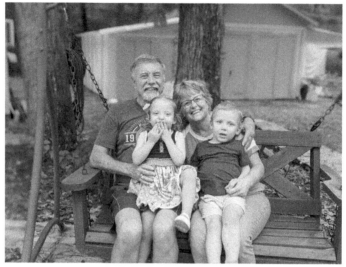

*Oliver & Kaylee with Beth and Larry Sparks at
their home during one of their many visits.*

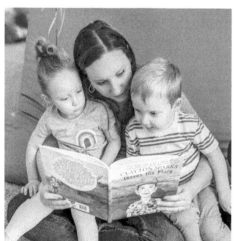

*Reading Clayton Sparks Leaves His
Mark to the kids. I love that they can
read this story about Clayton and
use it to spark kindness in others.*

*Each year as a family, we celebrate
Donate Life month in April and talk
about the importance of organ donation.*

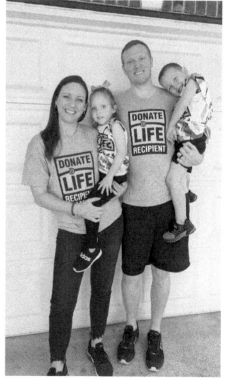

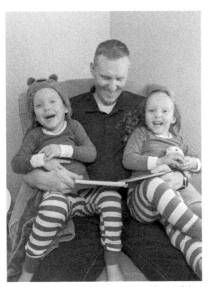

*Because of Clayton, Reid is able to read bedtime stories to Oliver and Kaylee each night.*

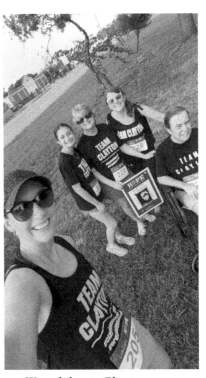

*We celebrate Clayton every chance we get. This was at the 2024 Second Chance Run benefiting LifeGift.*

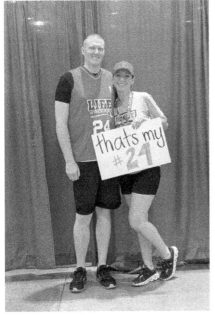

*Reid played basketball in the 2024 Transplant Games of America and took home a silver medal.*

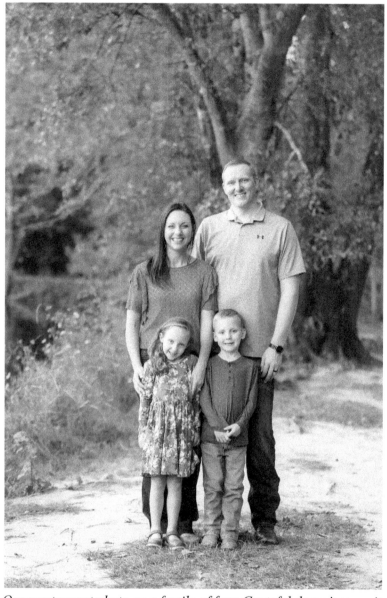

*Our most recent photo as a family of four. Grateful doesn't cover it.*

# Acknowledgements

**Reid,** thank you for always supporting me and whatever crazy idea I come up with. Not only did you agree with me putting our full story out there for the world to dissect, but you also spent hours reading and re-reading (and re-reading again) to make sure our story was captured in an impactful way. I appreciate that throughout our entire journey, your worry has always been *me*. You are an amazing husband and father; I am so grateful you are ours.

**Oliver & Kaylee,** there are no words to describe how deep my love for you both is. I know I won't ever be a perfect mom, but I hope you always know that I try my hardest for you. Don't ever lose sight of the miracles that exist in this world, and always take time to be grateful and soak in the little joys.

**Mom,** thank you for showing me from a young age what determination and drive look like. You and Dad both instilled a sense of professionalism and responsibility in me that I'm forever thankful for. Thank you for going above and beyond to ensure my husband was healthy and here for our children. I am forever grateful for you and the abundance of love you show us and everyone around you.

**Denise,** thank you for being there *literally* every step of the way. Thank you for sitting on the other end of the phone while I cried. Thank you for dropping everything in your busy life and being by my side when I needed you most. Thank you for being the person I can always count on, no matter what. "Best friend" doesn't accurately describe you; you're my soul sister.

**Tinker,** I truly won the jackpot having you and Ric as my in-laws. I know this entire journey filled you with so much worry and heartache. I am grateful for your steadfast support; you have always been there for everything we needed. Thank you for supporting my dream to share our full story with the world – and editing it so I sound like a better writer than I actually am. Thank you for raising the amazing man that you did. He is who he is because of you and Ric.

**Beth and Larry,** where do I even start? You came into our lives through organ donation, but our relationship has grown so much because of the amazing people that you both are. Not only did you take your immense grief and turn it into something beautiful for our family, you continue to pour so much love into us and the kids and I couldn't imagine our lives without the two of you. Oliver and Kaylee are incredibly blessed to have you as their BeBe and Pops.

**Dr. Griffith, Dr. Raijman, and Dr. Reddy,** you are all truly amazing human beings and the perfect example of how a doctor should treat their patients. The amount of love and support that you all showed us during the most difficult times of our lives is incredible. You all continued to fight for us and went above and beyond to help us see our miracles come to light.

**The Houston Methodist J.C. Walter Jr. Transplant Team,** I am forever grateful you saved my husband's life. I don't know exactly what happened in that OR the day of the transplant, and I don't know that I want to know. But I know it was a challenge, and I am so glad you all were there with him. I have no doubts that you all fought to keep my husband alive, and he is here for all of us as a result of your skills and determination. Thank you doesn't seem to be enough.

**Dad,** as much as I hated hearing you ask, "Now, what lesson did we learn from this?" growing up, I can appreciate the lessons you taught me now. I can look back at our entire journey and see all of the amazing growth opportunities and moments of hope. Thank you for helping me see that.

**My beta readers: Angie, Jessica, and Sarah,** You girls understood the assignment, and I appreciated every ounce of your feedback as you helped me make this book what it is today. All three of you spent an incredible amount of time helping me turn this project into something that would truly impact others. I'm so grateful you are all friends who can be honest with me and help me grow.

**Monroe,** I can't forget about my girl. You were there for some of the injections, but most importantly, you made me A&B cookies during our last round of IVF. You said at the time that the "A" was for "Abby" and "B" was for "Baby," but I think you secretly knew somehow I'd have a "Baby A" and "Baby B." Your cookies did the trick!

**Brenda,** thank you for being my publisher and friend. I'm so glad our paths crossed at just the right time. I'm incredibly grateful for your support and encouragement along the way.

**To our entire support system** – you know who you are, and there are way too many to name. We could not have gotten through this without all of you. Whether you realize it or not, you made a huge impact on us and were an incredible source of strength so we could keep fighting. I hope you continue to use our story to encourage others.

**My sweet Wrigley,** I hope you are running free in doggy heaven. You brought us so much joy during so many times of uncertainty. You were the best dog and I'm so grateful you were ours.

# About the Author

In January 2017, Abby Gray turned to writing as a therapeutic outlet. She started a blog when she and her husband, Reid, were navigating serious health challenges while trying to build a family. With Reid's ongoing health struggles, Abby found solace in her writing and the support of loved ones, creating a solid network of encouragement around her.

After four years of struggles, Abby and Reid experienced unexpected miracles that changed their lives in ways no one could have foreseen. Their remarkable journey has become one of hope and inspiration, and Abby feels called to share their story to bring hope to others facing similar struggles. She advocates passionately for organ donation, infertility awareness, and mental health and openly shares their experiences to help others find strength and encouragement.

In 2022, Abby released a children's book titled Clayton Sparks Leaves His Mark. The book encourages others to find ways to "spark" kindness, and gently opens up the conversation of organ donation within families.

Abby's mission can be summed up with these three words: Inspire. Engage. Connect.

More information and resources can be found at:

abbygraywrites.com